# THE COUCH OF
# WILLINGNESS

# THE COUCH OF WILLINGNESS

## AN ALCOHOLIC THERAPIST BATTLES THE BOTTLE AND A BROKEN RECOVERY SYSTEM

MICHAEL POND
AND
MAUREEN PALMER

Everywhere Now
www.everywherenowpress.com

**Library and Archives Canada Cataloguing in Publication**
Pond, Michael, 1953–, author
The couch of willingness: an alcoholic therapist battles the bottle and a broken recovery system / Michael Pond and Maureen Palmer.

ISBN 978-0-9937147-0-2 (pbk.)
ISBN 978-0-9937147-1-9

1. Pond, Michael, 1953–. 2. Alcoholics–British Columbia–Biography. 3. Psychotherapists–British Columbia–Biography. 4. Recovering alcoholics–British Columbia–Biography. 5. Alcoholics–Rehabilitation. 6. Alcoholism–Psychological aspects. 7. British Columbia–Biography. I. Palmer, Maureen, author II. Title.

HV5307.P66A3 2014          362.292092          C2014-901462-7

Cover design by Naomi MacDougall

*To my three sons: Taylor, Brennan and Jonathan, for allowing me to be their father again*

# CONTENTS

# PREFACE

I met Mike a few years ago on the dating website Plenty of Fish. On our first date he arrived on transit and ordered cranberry juice. Ashamed, he admitted he had lost his licence to drunk driving and had been sober just over a year. This is the part where my female friends screamed, "Run, run, run for the hills." Over the next few dates, Mike revealed such a riveting story, I blurted, "We have to write a book," to this near stranger. Initially, I was probably more intrigued with the story than the man. *The Couch of Willingness* is that story.

In telling this story, we needed to be respectful of people's privacy. Many names and other identifying information have been changed. This book is Mike Pond's truth. As much as possible, we corroborated events with others. We recently had coffee with Rhonda, Mike's ex-wife, who shook her head after reading the manuscript and said, "Mike, I can't believe how well you remembered all those horrible details, when you were so out of it!"

— Maureen Palmer

# 1

# THREE MILE BEACH

It's like a stuck record that no one nudges.

"Let me outta here! You sons of bitches! I wanna talk to my lawyer!" Dana's caterwauling reaches me from the solitary cell in the women's wing. It's getting on my nerves. It's three a.m. and she's been at it for hours.

"Cocksuckers. Let me talk to my lawyer. Let me out of here, you sons of bitches."

"Shut the fuck up, bitch!" another female inmate howls, matching Dana decibel for decibel. "I'm gonna fuck you up when we all get outta here, you drunken whore."

I roll over on the thin jail-cell pallet and pull the bleached blanket over my head in a useless attempt to drown out the hollering. I fade in and out of sleep, no longer able to discern what's a bad dream and what's an even worse reality.

I wish I'd never gone to Three Mile Beach.

The autumn sun's wan rays bathe everything at Three Mile Beach in light so fragile, so ephemeral, it's almost magical. A rare kind of day.

"Mr. Pond." Dana emerges from the lake, runs across the sand and stands before me glistening in the sun. "Let's move to Nelson and open up a treatment centre on Kootenay Lake.

It's our destiny. We are meant to do something amazing together."

I gaze into Dana's piercing blue eyes and I'm sick with longing. I long for her and the fantasy we've built together, a fantasy so flimsy I already feel it slipping away. She arranges her perfect coral-bikini-clad body on the towel, plants a kiss on my sun-burnished brow, lies down and closes her eyes. At forty-two, Dana's lithe, willowy beauty belies her age. I track a rivulet of water as it slides into the hollow between her breasts.

I'd always wanted to open a treatment centre. I'd been practising psychotherapy for over twenty years in Penticton, and I'd often thought I wouldn't have much of a practice at all if not for alcohol. From the surly conduct-disordered kid slouched on my couch to the shame-faced husband convicted of domestic assault, court-ordered into treatment, to the suicidal young First Nations mother of five kids, barely thirty and already worn out, you don't get too far in family-of-origin research before you stumble over a raging alcoholic. I'd helped hundreds of people kick booze. But I cannot help myself.

"Yeah, the universe has a grand plan for us, Dana." I try to muster enthusiasm as I lie back next to her. "We were put together to make great things happen." Great. Now I'm lying even to myself.

Dana exhales, her face breaking into a wide smile. Her perfect white teeth dazzle. I smell vodka. The fantasy fades just a little bit more.

Over the course of the afternoon at the beach, we polish off a twenty-sixer and a half of Smirnoff mixed with Clamato juice and a generous splash of Frank's hot sauce. We regale ourselves. We are as eloquent and witty and deep as only drunks can be.

Three Mile Beach edges Okanagan Lake in British

Columbia's hot, dry wine country. As Napa Valley is to California, the Okanagan is to Canada. Vines droop, burdened by lush late-harvest Gewürztraminer grapes, the air pungent with the earthy promise of ripe fruit. Vineyards march up every slope, stretching over the horizon, their uniformity broken here and there by the odd gnarled apple or pear tree, poignant reminders of the days when this was orchard country.

This is wine country, but we don't drink wine. One would have to drink too much and wait too long for its effect. Vodka is a much more efficient drunk. And after going hard at it for nearly a month, we are all about efficiency.

Forget wild sexual attraction, stimulating conversation, shared values and beliefs and interests. What keeps us together now is booze. Every encounter plays out in the same sickening sequence, from that first seductive sip to giddy intoxication, through belligerence and anger and exaggerated competence to melancholy and sullen self-pity, ending always in self-loathing.

Dana has just arrived at exaggerated competence.

"Mike, I want my kids to meet you." She gets up off her towel, brushing sand from her bare legs. "They're not far away, in Naramata. Let's go."

My judgment dulled by Smirnoff, I agree to this absurd idea. Who wouldn't want to meet mum's drunken boyfriend?

2

# THE VISIT

Dana drives deliberately slowly so as not to alert cops. The late-afternoon October sun still warms our shoulders as we crawl along in her little Miata. We first parallel the lake where sailboats dance on the sparkling water. Then we head along the mountain road below the old Kettle Valley rail bed to Naramata.

A tiny warning pings in my head.

"Dana, I don't think this is a good idea. Let's turn back, drop me off at my place."

"Oh no, I want them to meet you." Dana focuses on the road ahead. "I'm so proud of you."

I'm not proud of me. I'm a drunk.

We pull up to a 1960s two-storey and I'm filled with a sense of foreboding. Dana and her husband are separated, and her boys are living with their dad. He sounds like a pretty good guy. He lets Dana drop by to see her sons as much as she likes. I'm not sure how he'll feel about today's little unscheduled stop.

Dana slithers out of the driver's seat and staggers to the front door with me in tow. Her six-year-old son, just home from school, spies us first as we step into the house. He runs up and hugs Dana. Her older son walks in, and he and his brother exchange anxious here-we-go-again glances. The kids back away and sink simultaneously into the couch.

My presence seems to barely register, for which I am thankful. My stomach knots and my jaw clamps and my eyes dart around the room. I wish for a cloak of invisibility. I'm sobering up quickly, but Dana keeps kicking the vodka-and-orange back. She emerges from a bedroom, her drink mysteriously refreshed. She's got a stash everywhere. Under different circumstances, I consider that one of her greatest attributes.

Dana stands at the sink washing dishes, an intimately domestic task. All I can do is watch. I shouldn't be here. The children sit in a row on the couch, their eyes on the door, hoping for a miracle to walk in. Feigning nonchalance, I lean on the back of an old easy chair.

Finally, Dana's older son speaks in a tone and manner that children of alcoholics learn early. Don't want to set Mum off.

"Mum, maybe it would be better if you came back later?"

He and I lock eyes. I detect fear, disguised as anger. I look away.

"Dana, let's go," I urge. I take her by the elbow and guide her toward the door.

Too late. Dana's estranged husband appears in the doorway. He takes in the scene. I see on his face that odd blend of shock, resignation and the preternatural calm of those who love drunks.

Dana explodes.

"You useless prick." Her face contorts with rage. "I hate you."

Sean, clearly practised at this, sits down at the kitchen table. "Dana, you're drunk. Why don't you guys just leave?"

"You prick. You useless piece of shit," Dana spits.

Sean turns in his chair to face Dana and places both of his

hands on the table. The children scrunch closer together on the couch. Lizzy, an old white mutt, belly-crawls under the cherry coffee table, just her curlicue tail visible.

My mouth hangs open in shock. I have never heard my impeccable Dana talk this way.

"Dana, let's go." The fingers on my left hand embed into her upper arm flesh. "Let's get out of here."

With brute strength she wrenches free and lunges for the Henckels chef's knife on the kitchen counter.

"Not until I kill the bastard!" She wraps her elegant fingers around the black handle.

No time to process this lightning turn in Dana's personality — I jump to action.

"No, Mum, no!" Dana's son pleads from the couch. "Please just leave — just go!"

Sean grabs a kitchen chair and holds it between himself and Dana like a lion tamer. I dive for Dana, grab her wrist and wrench the knife from her hand.

"Let's just go, Dana. That's enough." I toss the knife back to the counter. I feel my carotid arteries pound.

Dana wrestles and kicks at me as I drag her out the door. They all stare after us, in part disbelief, part relief.

My mind reels. What the hell just happened? What happened to my beautiful Dana? Who is this woman?

I hear Sean on the phone behind us, talking to 911.

We bolt for what is now our getaway car. We jump in and Dana tears out of the driveway, spraying gravel everywhere, cursing vehemently at "the fucking male-dominated world" as we fishtail down the road. I can't take my eyes off her. I still can't quite believe she's the same person.

Though I'm closer to sober at this moment, Dana still has a driver's licence. Mine's been suspended. I picked up my first impaired driving charge a few months ago, at nine a.m. on my way to the liquor store. My second impaired charge came the very next day, also at nine a.m., on the way to the same liquor store. Then a few weeks ago I passed out at the wheel and slammed my brand-new Honda Ridgeline, the truck of my dreams, headlong into a wall of rock. It was my fifty-fifth birthday.

I'm riding shotgun for gawd-knows-how-long.

We careen through town in search of an escape route and squeal round the corner onto the highway. Her foot to the pedal, the sea-green Miata nose points ever higher up the steep slope. Dana is flushed, breathing rapidly and heavily, still trembling from the encounter with Sean. We climb and climb till the first bend, when Dana suddenly cranks the wheel right and the Miata heads east on an old dirt road toward the lake. We stop. There is no more road. Pumping the brakes, Dana nudges the nose of her car to the edge of a cliff.

The scene is surreal. Think Thelma and Louise in a British Columbia tourism ad. We teeter at the edge of the steep cliff overlooking Okanagan Lake. Dana's sports car perches precariously on the road edge, the ground beneath an unstable mix of sand, silt and gravel.

Two hundred feet below, the lake's shiny blue waters sparkle. A cloud of sandy dust and dirt drifts silently forward off the cliff. The sky fades from orange into purple. The sun sets.

Dana's manicured porcelain hands still grip the steering wheel. Her tousled hair hangs over her face. She blows away an out-of-place strand. Her bloodshot eyes glare straight ahead at nothing. They scare the shit out of me.

A few months ago, I fell in love with those eyes. It was a bright August day. I had taken my lunch break at Three Mile Beach. I was sitting staring out at the water, washing down my wrap with a Smirnoff cooler, when out of the corner of my eye I spied legs. Long, tanned legs. I tracked them up as they disappeared below a flimsy apple green sundress. She looked at me and smiled, then turned away with a bounce of her dark red curls. I watched her for the next few minutes. She kept glancing back.

I looked behind me to see if she was trying to make eye contact with someone there.

Nope. No one else on the beach.

I downed the last swig of the cooler and, with all the swagger a five-foot-six-inch guy can muster, I strode across the sand and introduced myself.

"Dana," she replied, and reached out to shake my hand.

She's getting divorced. She's moved up to the Okanagan from Vancouver. She's managing a friend's B & B. Two kids, living up here with her ex.

I commiserated. I too am getting a divorce, but I can't even get my act together to make that happen. We agreed to meet for coffee the next morning. That was the first and last coffee we shared. We immediately switched to the hard stuff. Dana is a drunk like me.

"Fuck." Dana squeezes the steering wheel. "I hate that prick. He called the cops."

The giddy, drunken exhilaration of being on the lam subsides. The gravity of our situation sinks in.

I need to take charge because I am closer to sober. I ease open the passenger door. I hate heights. I shuffle out of the car, leaning back as if leaning forward would send me cascading over the edge. I peer down just enough to see the lake. I edge back and around the car to the driver's side and swing open the door.

"Get out. I'm driving. You're going to kill someone."

"No. Fuck off. I'm driving. I still have a licence, you prick." Dana stares out the windshield.

How did I so quickly become the prick?

I shove her toward the passenger side. She slides over,

glances sulkily my way then out the window. I climb into the driver's seat, press the brake, rev the Miata in reverse, back away from the cliff edge and turn the car around. We don't get far before I hear it. The faint wail of police sirens echo up the valley.

As I round the first bend, the wail accelerates and amplifies. I squint in the rear-view mirror to see three RCMP cruisers closing on us, really fast. Should I try to outrun them?

Sober second thought intervenes. I pull over.

The officers haul us out, splay us spread-eagled over the trunk of a patrol car and pat search, and then not-so-gently handcuff us. I am subdued, fearful and aghast, a star in my own getaway movie. Dana wriggles, fights, slips a hand out of the cuffs and whoops in triumph. "Did you see that, you fucking pricks!" She pumps her liberated fist into the clear night sky.

Her bravado doesn't last long. Cops quickly re-cuff her, tighter now, and dip her head into the back seat of the first car. I get ducked into the second car, and the third cruiser brings up the rear. As we pull out onto the highway, I can still hear Dana screaming. We head back to the Penticton drunk tank.

## 3

# BONNIE AND CLYDE GO TO JAIL

Frank is the processing officer tonight. Shit. We played on the same hockey team. Our sons played hockey together since they were toddlers. Countless times over countless beers, we've engaged in play-by-play analysis of the boys' games. We've bunked together on tournament trips. Played poker into the wee hours of the night, carrying on like old buddies. We *are* old buddies.

Tonight, Frank is all business. He ushers me in to the back room. Sits me down in front of the Breathalyzer. With resignation, I blow. He and I both know I'm over the legal limit — by a lot. He takes my fingerprints, then my mug shot. As he fills in the requisite forms, Frank pauses and peers at me.

"Please get some help, Mike." His pen hovers over the form. "You've got to stop. You're needed in this community."

"Thanks, Frank, I will." I hang my aching head. I know I won't. Not today, anyway. I need a drink.

Eyes down, I shuffle into my cell. The door slams behind me. A sour stench assaults my nose — a blend of vomit, bleach, urine and sweat. I shake and my stomach lurches. I hurl myself toward the standard jail-issue stainless steel toilet and just make it. I wretch and vomit and wretch and vomit and dry heave again and again and again until I stop and lie spent on the concrete floor beside the toilet. In just a few hours, blessed dawn will save me from this fetid hole. We'll get sprung, the liquor store will open, I'll get my medicine and the shakes will stop.

I peel myself off the floor and collapse onto the bed, cold, battleship-grey painted metal with a one-and-a-half-inch-thick black plastic mat like the ones you use at the gym to do sit-ups. I pull the blanket over my aching body, aware of the rush of red heat up the sides of my neck delivering guilt, shame, recrimination and the inevitable self-loathing.

With most of the alcohol purged from my system, I contemplate this disastrous turn of events. Dana is charged with uttering threats. I have a third impaired driving charge. *Three* impaired driving charges! I could have killed someone. When working with clients who've driven drunk, I've always dispassionately wondered how in this day and age anyone could drive drunk.

Now I know.

How will I ever look my three sons in the eye, especially Taylor, my oldest? He took on the burden of preventing me from driving drunk. He developed a sixth sense, anticipating that moment before the alcoholic's judgment gives out and the grandiose sense of self kicks in. That very last moment when I still had a single shred of good sense, he'd show up and demand I hand over my car keys. A few days later he'd show up and hand them back, knowing he'd have to do it all over again in another few days. The last time he knocked on my door, I was deep in DTs, detoxing, and he sat at the foot of my bed for forty-eight hours to see me through it.

"It's gonna be okay, Dad. You're gonna get through this. You need some Tylenol? I'll get you some more water."

Once healthy enough to walk, in a swift betrayal of his

compassion I immediately shuffled down to Bubblees, my favourite liquor store, right next door to the local peeler bar, Slack Alice's, and stocked up on Smirnoff. Back home, when I was deep into my bender, Taylor showed up, a moment too late this time. I was on top of my game, impervious. There was nothing I couldn't do. I refused to hand over the keys. He wrestled them from my hands, then stared at me. Something in his eyes changed. He tossed the keys on the kitchen counter and walked out the door.

Not so long ago, my three boys were the centre of my life. I loved being a dad. Back in 1992, after work I'd rush home in the early winter twilight and head directly to the backyard, grab the pistol nozzle of the crackling stiff green garden hose and stand there for hours, night after night, flooding layer after layer, letting each layer freeze until the sheet of ice shone smooth like black glass in the moonlight. I constructed the rink boards with two-by-fours and four-by-eight sheets of half-inch Douglas fir plywood to create two-foot-high walls around the rink that took up almost the entire backyard. We called it "The Forum." I installed floodlights at each end. Then Team Pond took on all comers. Seven-year-old Taylor already had the style and confidence of a pro. Five-year-old Brennie attacked the puck with gritty determination. And three-year-old Jonny, well, he was so cute all he had to do was show up. I was player, coach, trainer, manager, first-aid attendant, water boy and referee. Brennan argued every call I made. Time suspended as we perfected passes, pretended to be Gretzky, Lemieux, Orr and Lafleur. And we always beat the Bruins for the Stanley Cup. My wife, Rhonda, good-natured but exasperated, would yell herself hoarse. "All right, you guys, that's enough. Mike, the boys have to come in. It's way past their bedtime."

Regret.

I'm probably going to jail, where I belong. Quickly now

before I forget ... Thank you, dear God, for saving me from killing someone, for keeping an eye on me when everyone else has given up the job.

More incomprehensible shrieks from Dana interrupt my reverie. I hear the overnight duty officer reprimand her.

"Ma'am, stop pushing your feet through the food slot. Please remove your feet."

I envision her pretty red-painted toes protruding through the food slot. How did this get to be my life?

Who will see my clients when I'm in jail? With all my drunk-driving infractions, I'll lose my driver's licence for life. And worse, I'll lose my licence to practise psychotherapy.

My hands vibrate. I'm going to be sick again.


The police release us at 8:37 the next morning. Twenty-three unbearably long minutes until a liquor store opens. The car impounded, we walk arm in arm, more to hold each other up than out of affection, to the nearest liquor store, in Penticton Plaza at Main and Duncan. We sit in silence on the curb in front of the liquor store. It's not cold, but we both shiver. Shoppers heading into Safeway shoot condemning looks our way.

Someday soon, we'll have our day in court. But today the party continues.

The young clerk can't quite hide his disdain as he rings in another forty-pounder. We're past caring. We take a cab to the dilapidated little bungalow that I share with brain-injured Todd. A friend who knew I was down on my luck — and knew Todd needed company — suggested we bunk together. His house is within two blocks of three liquor stores, the home that is a metaphor for what has become of my life.

# 4

# GETTING HERE

My life has shrunk to a radius of about eight blocks of down-town Penticton that stretches from this little cottage that I share with Todd on Government Street to my office over on Main Street. My office, where I still have the audacity to see clients. Without a car, without a licence, I ride — no, wobble — to work on my bike through Penticton's back alleys. If I stick to the back alleys, no one will know that I drink.

Earlier this summer I was weaving down the back alley behind my office, helmet dangling from the handlebars, clutching a bottle of Smirnoff in one hand, when a familiar young voice called out to me.

"Hey, Mr. Pond, is that you?"

I foot-stomped my bike to a shaky stop by the dumpster behind Martinis, a new nightclub on Martin Street. Careful. Don't drop the bottle. The bike stopped with a chainy clunk.

"Hey, Bryce, how you doing?" I steadied myself and tried to look nonchalant.

"Mr. Pond ... that you?" Bryce played minor hockey with my oldest son for years. Emotions fast-forwarded across his face. Shock gave way to pity gave way to concern gave way to embarrassment. I had to get out of here.

"Everything's great," I yelled as I pushed off and rode, pumping furiously past him. "I'm late for a client," I yelled over my shoulder. I looked down at my feet. I had only one shoe on.

There's a photo of me from the day I got my master's of social work, beaming proudly, surrounded by my equally proud mum and family. The boys were very young when I decided to go back to school. Nights I pulled the graveyard shift at Juvenile Services to the Courts. Days I spent at the University of British Columbia in Vancouver, cramming my sleep-deprived brain full of Adler, Ellis and Jung. So tired ... I remember waking up toward the end of that year with a start, hands gripped white on the steering wheel in the dark and drizzly pre-dawn. The transport in my lane blasted his horn. Then the sick realization: I'm in *his*. He careened over to the shoulder and saved both our lives.

Back then I drank only on weekends, when all the other young fathers did. Never wavered. Some kind of subconscious survival strategy looped in my brain: "Drink during the week now, buddy, and you are done."

But as thesis time approached I could not keep up with the punishing workload. On the final weekend, the thesis due on Monday morning, I wrote around the clock. Up in the kitchen cupboard, tucked in the back of my mind: a full bottle of Bacardi white rum. Sunday at noon it whispered to me. I ignored it. By ten p.m. I was positively vibrating with anxiety and anticipation. With the boys and Rhonda in bed, I clamoured to the cupboard and broke the seal, and the booze and the prose flowed. I finished the bottle — and the thesis — off at five Monday morning. I fell asleep on the couch. Rhonda quietly got the boys up and hushed them off to school, where she worked as a teaching assistant.

Almost noon I woke up to find the empty bottle of Bacardi tucked in beside me on the couch. I wrenched it out with a little too much force and it flung past me to shatter on the floor. Shit. Shards everywhere. I rushed to pick them up, cutting my feet in the dash to the kitchen for the dustpan. Blood gushed and puddled on the floor and oozed out over the edge of the white dining-room carpet. I felt woozy and sank down again on the couch.

I woke up next sure that someone was watching me. Glanced at the clock. Holy shit — it was three thirty. The kids were due home from school any minute. But it was too late. Ten-year-old Taylor stood at the end of the couch and looked at me, confused and afraid. "Are you okay, Dad? There's blood on your feet. And there's some on the carpet."

"Yeah, I'm not feeling very good, and I accidentally broke a glass. It's okay. You go upstairs and play."

I cleaned up the mess before Rhonda got home with the younger boys, then, riddled with guilt, I took Taylor to McDonald's. And as he stuffed a Big Mac in his mouth, I talked.

"Did it scare you when you saw me like that?"

"Yeah, Dad, it did. It scares me when you get drunk."

"It will never happen again, Tay. I promise. I don't want to scare you or your brothers. Or your mum." I hugged him, softly rubbed his back and tousled his head of blond curls. "I love you, son."

We chowed down our meal and I vowed to myself that this had been my last bender.

When we got home, I resolutely told a relieved Rhonda, "I'm going to AA."

Passing out in front of Taylor scared me into action.

I went to my first AA meeting. But I wasn't like those people. They were drunks. I sat through the entire meeting without saying a word. As I left, an old fellow said, "If yer thinkin' 'bout drinkin' or thinkin' 'bout not drinkin', yer an alcoholic." I didn't want to admit yet just how much my thinking revolved around drinking.

In 1995 I got my master's. We returned to Penticton. I quit my government job, cashed in my pension to set up my private practice. "Stay the course, Michael," was the audio loop that played now. Every time I felt the urge to drink, I went mountain biking or played hockey. Or snowboarded with the boys. Or worked more.

In 1996 the practice took off. Each successful relationship built with a client begat several more. By 2000, after a few years of favourable word of mouth, the agencies came calling. Workers' Compensation. Health Canada. The Insurance Corporation of British Columbia. The RCMP's Victim Services. The school boards. The Indian bands.

Lucrative contracts meant I could hire staff. At my peak in the early 2000s, we had four counsellors and an office manager working for Michael Pond Associates Ltd.

As the business boomed, so did our social life, which swirled around hockey. Every day the boys practised or had games. I played three times a week with my buddies, most of us dads with our kids in Minor Hockey. After games, we'd all go for beers and nachos at the Barking Parrot or the Barley Mill.

Weekends shifted to the boys' games. Cradling beers, all the dads screamed support to their sons and heckled refs.

"Put your whistle in your pocket!"

"Get some glasses, ref!"

"Homer!"

After the game, the partying moved to a designated house — often ours. As a dozen young boys careened around the house, their parents got plastered. Three beers became four. I'm not alone in excess. We all drink too much, laugh too loud. We egg each other on. "C'mon, Mike, have a rum and Coke." "Hey, try this new martini." Every winter weekend becomes a socially sanctioned bender.

When summer arrived, we switched to barbecues. Living

in the heart of wine country, Friday-Saturday-Sunday became one extended wine tasting. Friends who worked in the industry introduced us to each new varietal. Everyone else sipped. But as time progressed, I pounded them back. I drank faster than everyone else and consumed a lot more. "Oh, Mike, you were so funny last night" became "It's nine thirty and there's Pond, passed out on the couch again."

But during weekdays, I still function. Up at five a.m., take the boys to hockey, go for a bike ride, office by seven, do reports and invoices, see clients, go home, enjoy a rum and Coke with Rhonda, put the kids to bed, have a few more rum and Cokes. Hey, I can handle this.

2001. More warning signs. I began to create little stashes of gin in the garage, on the new boat. In the summer of 2002 I counted at least twenty "wine-tasting" parties. I'd go to the parties then come home and hit my stashes. The audio loop was now "Hey, buddy, don't you think you better cut back?" But I don't want to stop. I can't stop. Alcohol is woven into everything that gives my life meaning. My boys' sports. My evenings kicking back with rum and Coke and Rhonda. The warmth, the security of belonging to a tight-knit group of friends, intimacies shared, relationships forged over successive glasses of wine. Can you think of a worse place in Canada to live for an alcoholic than the Okanagan? How many times did Rhonda and I mix up gin and tonics and cart our lawn chairs down to the shore of Skaha Lake to watch the sun set? I can't give that up.

As my drinking ramps up, my practice is increasingly focused on dealing with alcohol's devastating impact. I sit on two boards for Victim Services and the Brain Injury Society and counsel those who've survived catastrophic crashes where a drunk was at the wheel. I look down at my notes. At one meeting my hand is vibrating so badly I can't read my own handwriting.

Referrals from the Ministry for Children and Family Development bring broken families, many of them First Nations, often involving child sexual abuse. My thesis had been a treatment outcome study of adolescent sex offenders, so I was well equipped to deal with this kind of trauma. Or so I thought.

The more I work with the First Nations families, the more I see how endemic sexual abuse is. Standard family-of-origin intake histories reveal abusers and abused in every generation. We don't understand this yet, but this is the brutal legacy of life in residential schools, a legacy that never touches non-Aboriginals except when the tragic headlines leap out of the morning paper.

"Teen runs over her own brother on local reserve." "Three brothers under 15 burn to death in teepee fire." "First Nations youth shoots his own cousins in drunken drug war." We ingest the latest horror with astounding indifference.

"Critical incident stress management." That's what I did. I'd be called to the charred remains of the teepee, where chaos reigned, where the sound of ceremonial drumming, keening and wailing punctuated by screaming condemnation filled the early-morning winter air. I'd attempt to soothe the unsoothable. I'd book follow-up appointments for grieving family members and the RCMP officer first upon the grisly scene.

Then I'd get back in my truck and drive back over the mountain, and in the solitude and quiet, the tears would come. I'd unconsciously drive to the nearest bar and pound back a shooter, look down and my hands would be shaking again. The next day there would be a dozen angry phone calls. People threatening to kill people. But each time on the way home, there was this little window of time where the warmth of the booze took the edge off. "How can I hold it together?" I asked myself. Over and over.

I didn't.

The superintendent of the school district gave me several warnings then pulled my contract.

One of the school counsellors said, "Mike, you're more fucked up than the families we send to you. Get help."

A client from one of my Employee Assistance Program contracts came to my office and knocked on the door. I heard her. I lay on my couch, sick with detoxing and so hungover I couldn't possibly respond. She knocked over and over and over and finally I staggered to the door and flung it open. "Oh my God, you've been drinking," she said. She fled.

Rhonda wanted me to cut back. She got ever more insistent. First I tried the controlled drinking model. I knew the literature said it rarely works. "Okay, Rhonda, at the barbecue I'm only going to have two beers." I'd be on beer number one and one of the guys would walk by and say, "Here, Mike, try this new spiced rum." Or, "Pond, you're the only one who didn't get a shooter. Push this one back." Rhonda would cruise past, see the beer in my hand and say, "Is that still your first beer?"

"Yes it is." But Rhonda's no fool.

I began to call in sick, telling my staff to cancel all my clients and reschedule. "I have the flu."

I'd get up after a day or two and still be half-loaded. Couldn't go in. Called my staff again and told them to cancel and reschedule again. And again.

One night I broke down the two doors to my office because I needed a place to sleep. An early-morning client walked in through the smashed-in door frames and found me passed out on the leather sectional. The next day, four resignations sat lined up on my desk. All the staff had quit. "Mike, I'm not going to cover up for you anymore."

Then it became Rhonda's job. She couldn't do it either.

So I promised to stop. Again.

I tried abstinence. I can quit drinking, I said to myself. I did. Dozens of times over 2003, 2004 and 2005. I'd stay dry for a couple of weeks at the most. Once I made it three months. Then I took the boys on an idyllic snowboarding weekend at Sun Peaks Resort. I dropped them off at their friends' and started to feel sad. Overwhelmed by all the damage I'd done to my relationship with my sons because of my drinking, what did I do? I got drunk.

In 2005 Rhonda and I did a $125,000 renovation to our home on the shores of Skaha Lake. The two-storey lakeside house now looks like the big reveal on some TV makeover show. The entire north wall is gone, replaced with an expanse of elegant French doors that open to a pressed concrete patio, where a soft waterfall spills into a rock pond. Inside, solid black walnut floors stretch the length of the house. But the kitchen — oh, that kitchen! That's where we blew the wad. The custom-designed, custom-built cabinets. The centrepiece: a black granite-topped custom-built island. Above it, light fixtures from a high-end design store in Vancouver's swank South Granville shopping area. Nine hundred fifty dollars each. At my count that's about forty bottles of Smirnoff. The sad irony: Now that I have the house I always dreamed about, I'm no longer welcome in it.

My last day in the house: I'm laid out corpse-like on Jonny's bed. The ratty bent venetian blinds, closed tight, bang tinnily on the taupe windowsill in rhythm with the cold wind blowing off the lake. The plastic bell-shaped ends of the pull strings tapped against the taupe wall, and that chocolate lab down the street barks.

Sick and shaky, I stare up at fluorescent stickers of little moons and stars that burnt out long ago. Jonny was five when he and his brothers stuck them on the ceilings of their bedrooms. Holed up now for four days of hard and heavy drinking, I pull back the beige and dark brown faux-suede comforter that smells like Jonny — that combo of young teenager high-energy sweat and warm sleep-tousled hair. I survey the room, almost as if I know I am taking it in for the last time. The closet, jammed with snowboard boots and hard-worn runners; broken skateboards and a toolbox-sized Samsung ghetto blaster piled up the wall; the broken sliding closet door, hanging by one brass hinge. I meant to fix that in the summer. Hoodies, T-shirts and frayed-hem jeans thrown high on top of the chipped blue dresser. And just out of reach on the floor, five empty vodka bottles. Jonny was sleeping in Taylor's room. He didn't want to see me or talk to me.

An abrupt, angry triple knock on the door lifted my splitting head off the bed. Rhonda stood by the open door, arm outstretched, her hand clamped on the doorknob. I could see the dark brown dime-sized birthmark on the top of her right wrist. It has always charmed me, ever since we first met in the summer of '82 at Bridges Restaurant on Granville Island.

"You have to leave, Mike." Her voice shook. "The boys and I have had enough. You've been holed up here drinking for four days."

When I first met Rhonda, I fell in love with her classic beauty. Big, striking deep blue eyes framed by long, full lashes. Strong Nordic features — a classic nose and that tiny cleft in her chin — and a shampoo commercial full of dark sexy curls. Everyone thought she was a model: tall and gorgeous. At almost six feet, she towered over me, but I didn't care. And to my immense good fortune, neither did she.

That day in Jonny's room, her elegant frame looked shrunken, hunched and defeated in the doorway. Her eyes showed that she'd gone past hurt and disappointment to something even more frightening — indifference.

"I know. I'll leave right away." My mouth, dry and gritty, choked on the words.

"Do you know what you're doing to your sons? Do you know what you're doing to me?"

"I'm sorry, Rhonda. I will stop." I coughed.

As if she hadn't heard me, Rhonda pulled the door closed.

"Just go, Mike. I don't care anymore." The door clicked shut.

I packed a small bag with toiletries, underwear, socks and one change of clothes and drove slowly to the Slumber Lodge Motel, where for weeks I faded in and out of an alcoholic fog just enough to hear the sounds of summer life echo across the water. Children's laughter. Dogs barking. Tunes and chatter from the multitude of boats cruising Lake Okanagan. The intimate murmurs and soft giggles of courting couples. I knew life was passing me by, and there wasn't a damn thing I could do about it. I told myself, this is temporary. She'll take me back.

That was almost three years ago.

I no longer waste energy bothering to keep up appearances. I just want to hole up with my girlfriend and get drunk. After our night in the drunk tank, in the tiny kitchen of Todd's little bungalow, Dana and I create a variety of vodka-based concoctions. Caesars made with extra hot and spicy Clamato juice and pickled asparagus stir sticks. Screwdrivers made with hand-squeezed orange juice. Black Russians made with Rockstar Coffee Energy Drink. Smirnoff's Ice Coolers enhanced with a couple of added shots. We gulp down our cocktails as if they were soda pop. I try to make eye contact with Dana. She looks at me but doesn't see me. I stare into her eyes hoping to make a connection. Those eyes look back at me, empty. It's a familiar look. I've seen it before in the empty blue eyes of my father.

## 5

# SANDY LAKE

Shilo is a small army base in southern Manitoba, about a two-hour drive west of Winnipeg and forty-five minutes north of the North Dakota border. It's smack dab in the middle of the vast plains that stretch across the continent. "Fly-over country," sophisticated East Coasters like to call it. We live at #39 Kingston Avenue. Ours is a small four-bedroom, two-storey duplex with a green plastic-coated clothesline running the length of the yard from the back doorway. Mum hangs clothes winter and summer. I help her take off the frozen sheets and towels, stiff boards of linen and terrycloth.

On this early summer day in 1965, Mum is in the hospital for an operation. "Women's stuff," says Dad. She isn't gone a day and my dad is on a bad drunk. He staggers around the house, giving us orders.

"Michael, pack us enough stuff for a few days for you, Roger and the girls," he slurs. "We can go fishing and just relax while your mother's in the hospital."

"I don't think that's a good idea, Dad. Why don't we just stay home and we can pitch the tent in the backyard." I want to distract him. Make him think about something else, anything to derail a disaster. I know these plans. I've been in on a lot of them.

Going hunting drunk. Going fishing drunk. Flying the plane drunk. Driving to hockey drunk.

Today's grand plan is to go away to a cabin at Sandy Lake, about ninety miles north, for a fun family holiday. The four of us kids look at each other, hoping someone will run for it. The rest would follow. We are all close to two years apart. I'm the oldest, at eleven. Then Roger, ten, Loretta, eight, and Danette, five. I'm used to running the household, but today I just don't have the energy to lead a mutiny.

I ache with familiar doubt. My stomach hurts and my face burns. My legs and jaw stiffen.

We half-heartedly pack the '64 Guardsman blue Mercury Comet Caliente. The car is always tuned up and the oil always changed. Dad is in the Royal Canadian Electrical Mechanical Engineers. "Change the oil regularly and keep her tuned up and your vehicle will last forever, especially a Ford," he once told me.

Dad loves Fords. And Volkswagens. "That Ford 289 V8 ... best engine ever designed. But the Krauts, they make the best vehicles." Dad says they're geniuses when it comes to anything mechanical.

"Those square-heads are smart and damn hard workers. Just don't buy anything the Japs make. They're sneaky little sons a' whores. Look what they did at Pearl Harbor."

We arrive at Sandy Lake late in the day. It's a small resort town with a soft beach and lots of perch and pickerel. Little summer cabins dot the shore. As we pass through the town, I spot a small hotel with a bar.

Several Indians loiter out front drinking beer and smoking cigarettes. A couple of doors down, by the post office, I see a small grocery store. Dad's eyes follow the hotel as we pass by on our way to the cabin. About a mile out of town, Dad pulls into a tiny driveway leading to our cabin, one of those dots on the lake.

A small, well-made dock stretches from the backyard right over the water. My little sisters jump out and dash to the end of the dock. They drop down to their knees, peer into the clear water and exclaim, "Hey, look! There's a whole bunch of little yellow fish! Mike, can we go fishing?"

Dad says, "Those are perch. Good eatin', but bony."

We scramble to bring our stuff in. I make the bed assignments. The beds are small, even by kid standards. A vague musty smell hangs in the air.

"I'm going into town to get some groceries for dinner and some fishing gear," Dad says. "You kids make a fire in the stove and play down at the beach."

He looks down at me. "Michael, look after things and I'll be back in a bit." And he leaves.

This is not the first time I've been told to "look after things." At twelve, I am mature beyond my years. Partly because every time Dad has gone on a bender, I've "manned up" for Mum. But mostly because I figured out the only way to survive as the shortest person in my school is to assume a leadership position.

I wanted to play hockey, so I had to skate faster than the rest. My punches had to land harder. I made the team. I also made the football team, but they didn't have pants small enough, so a football mum made the necessary adjustments. We were playing the team from Carberry, Manitoba, all corn-fed six-foot strapping Scandinavian farm boys, a team of giants. One tried to tackle me, but I was so fast he missed me and grabbed my pants, which ripped off. I scored a touchdown in my jock. I was also the high-jump champion, to the disbelief of my classmates. Held the record for years, so I'm told. All of which is my way of saying I learned early the importance of perseverance and determination, of sticking up for myself. "Bitesize. Shorty. Half-a-Man. Little Fella.

Shrimp." The nicknames stuck, said now with warmth and respect, the sting gone.

I fashion us all fishing rods out of willow branches and some old line and hooks I find in a broom closet by the wood stove. The fire in the stove sputters and hisses.

"Michael, Michael, take us down to fish," my little sisters beg. I turn the little cottage upside down, but there is no bait to be found, and no shovel to dig for worms. I improvise with a soup ladle and fail miserably.

Finally, my brother Roger's face lights up. "Let's try my Silly Putty," he grins. We put a little gob on each of our hooks. The perch love it. Stupid fish. As the warm summer afternoon wears on, we fish and we fish. Big fat horseflies drone in the background, occasionally swooping in for the kill. Our noses turned bright pink. Our freckles pop. Between us we catch eleven pretty little perch, all about four to six inches long. They'd taste great fried in butter. If only we had butter.

The air is still warm as the shadows lengthen and the sun glints lower now through the shimmering poplar trees. I ache for Mum. She'd fry up those little fish in no time.

"Michael, I'm hungry. I'm tired. When can we eat?" Danette whines.

"Can you cook our fish, Michael?" Loretta asks.

I know what I have to do. "Rog, keep an eye on Loretta and Danette. Don't let them down by the water. I'm gonna get Dad."

As fast as my short legs will carry me, I beeline for the hotel bar. I hear it before I see it. I hesitate at the door. With a deep breath, I shove it open.

Dad sits at a red terry-covered round table laughing, with a shorty beer bottle in his hand. A Native woman snuggles on his lap. I walk over to him. He glances past me, then his head whips back.

"Michael," he says in a low voice. "You're not supposed to be here. Go back to the cabin, I'll be there in a bit."

I stomp outside and wait on the curb by the hotel. And wait. And wait. It's dark now and I worry about the kids. With a goodbye glance at the well-worn bar door, I trudge back to the cabin.

The kids sit together at the kitchen table playing Snakes and Ladders.

"Mike, we're hungry," says Loretta. "Where's Dad?"

I don't answer. Instead, I wordlessly gut, clean and fry the perch.

We devour them. They are delicious, even without butter. Satiated, now sleepy, I tuck the little girls into bed in one small room, then Roger and I take the small bed in the other. We're just about asleep when I hear loud bangs.

Bodies lurch and sway in search of balance, knocking over furniture. I peer out the curtain that hangs in the doorway to our little room. There's Dad, stumbling in. Outside, Hank Snow sings "I'm Moving On" from the radio in the Comet.

Here comes an Indian couple. Then a man dressed in jeans, cowboy boots and a straw cowboy hat. They all smoke cigarettes and the men each carry a case of beer. This party is just getting started.

I want with all my heart to tell Dad and his new-found friends to get the hell out. I fall back asleep as Hank croons away. I wake up as the cowboy crawls into the small bed with my brother and me, still wearing his hat and boots. He stinks of stale beer, cigarettes, cow shit and BO. He slips his arm around my neck.

I slide out of the cot onto the cold floor, leaving Rog in the bed with this stranger who stinks.

Eyes wide open now, I hear the sounds of sex. It won't

stop. I hate to look, afraid of what I might see, but I have to look.

I peek into the living room and see Dad on the dingy brown couch with the Indian woman. Hatred flares up from my gut, sears my brain. The Native man is passed out in a chair, oblivious or desensitized or both.

I wonder about Mum in the hospital and hope she's okay.

I lie back on the cold floor. I just want to take the kids and go home. I know how to drive. It would be easy. But I just lie there until it's quiet, other than the incessant snoring of the cowboy. His arm is around Rog now. I feel like killing somebody. Eventually, I fall asleep.

When I wake up, everyone is gone — everyone but Dad. He sits at the little kitchen table. That look: I've seen it so many times by now. Is it guilt? Remorse?

No. It's a hangover. Leftover drunkenness and self-pity. He looks at me, those blue eyes empty.

"I gotta go to the store and get us some grub," Dad mutters. "Take care of your brother and sisters. I'll be back in a bit."

I look after him in disgust. I think: When I grow up, I'll never drink like him.

# 6

# COME DOWN HERE, MR. POND

Well, here I am: all grown up. There's an empty forty-pounder on the night table, and now I'm exactly like him. After two weeks of binge drinking at Todd's, there's not a drop left in the house. My hand rests in a soft indentation on the side of the bed where Dana should be. Every time I pass out, she disappears. I get up and stumble to the bathroom. I hear the TV down in the basement. Whenever we get rollin' on the booze, Todd retreats to the basement. I swing open the front door to get a breath of the cool, crisp fall air.

How long since Dana left? I have no idea.

Plates littered with shards of burnt toast and hardened egg yolk ring my bed. I need a drink. I slink down the stairs into Todd's tiny windowless, airless bedroom. I tiptoe my way through piles of stale, dirty laundry. I don't turn the light on — don't want to alert him to my presence. I hear him laugh at the TV. Good. I rummage through the collection of rolled quarters and loonies Todd keeps on his dresser in an old tattered basket. Many times I've helped him roll his spare change while we sat watching the hockey game. Twenty years ago, Todd was robbed and smashed in the head with a two-by-four, which left him permanently brain-damaged. Now he's being robbed again.

I sneak back upstairs. The phone rings. I recognize the number. It's Dana's sister's, in Vancouver.

"Come down here, Mr. Pond," Dana's voice sounds heavy and sad. "I'm not doing very well. I need you, Mr. Pond. Please, please, you have to come and help me."

I hang up the phone. Dana needs me. How many loonies for the six-hour bus ride to Vancouver?

"This is the last stop, buddy, you have to get off." The bus driver shakes me awake. When he turns his back, I gulp the last few ounces of vodka from the bottle stowed in my backpack, bought with Todd's rolled quarters. Outside in the cold late-October rain, the driver hoists my duffle bag out of the underside baggage compartment and watches me, somewhat concerned. Stiff and wobbly, I collect my wet bag and pour myself out into the heart of Vancouver's notorious Downtown Eastside.

I've got to call Dana. I need to find a payphone, because I left my cell in Dana's Miata, now in the impound lot in Penticton.

And — holy shit! — that's not all we forgot. I slap my forehead. The synapses all firing now, I remember: there's a hundred pounds of moose meat in the trunk, too.

Before the binge at Todd's, I'd been out hunting with First Nations friends, and a cache of cut and wrapped meat had been loaded into Dana's trunk. That was two weeks ago. They'll have pried open the trunk by now, convinced there's a body in it.

I giggle to myself. Down here, this kind of behaviour doesn't get a glance.

After the warmth of the Okanagan, the coast's cold rain feels like an assault. Heavy winds whip the water sideways. It lashes the near-deserted streets and pounds so hard that the drains, blocked by decaying leaves, can't keep up. In the dark and in my drunken state, I can't dodge the dozens of ankle-deep puddles. My socks squelch in my shoes. As I lurch from door to door, I find every covered stoop already spoken for. The godforsaken wretches down here have one up on me — they know the lay of the land.

At least I have a warm bed to go to, with a warm woman waiting. Finally, I spy a payphone.

The last payphone on the Downtown Eastside is my salvation. Even the druggies have cellphones now. I squeeze into the booth and shut the door against the wind and rain. I keep one eye trained on my duffle bag, as it now holds all my worldly possessions. Dana's cell goes directly to voice mail. She probably lost her cell. Again.

I dial Dana's sister's number collect. 604-267-3 ... 604-268-2 ... No, that's not it. I jab the keys. My panic mounts. I pound every permutation. I try dozens of numbers. None is Dana's sister's — a number I have dialled dozens of times but that I cannot remember.

I'm stone cold sober now. I need a drink. But I have no money.

Gentrification has crept into Vancouver's Downtown Eastside. Well-heeled diners sidestep massive puddles and run the gauntlet of shopping carts to line up in front of the latest hot restaurant. They glance in my direction but my presence barely registers. My cloak of invisibility finally seems to be working. More seasoned entrepreneurial drunks and addicts offer to hold the diners' places in line, save their parking spots, watch their cars.

As I round a familiar corner, loud, thumping music drifts from a club. When I first arrived in Vancouver some thirty years ago, I probably patronized this place myself.

I have no money, a concept I can't quite get my head

around. "No money" used to mean, just pull out a credit card. Mine are all suspended for non-payment. My one remaining bank account — joint — Rhonda has justifiably frozen.

A rush of blood, heat, races up the sides of my neck, and my face flushes a fiery red shame. I look down at my feet, put my hand out and mumble to the kind of people I used to be. "Do you have any spare change?" I look down to the shaking hand. That can't be my hand.

I can't make eye contact. I can't be aggressive. I can't do it. I'm a failure at panhandling.

The craving for vodka courses through my veins. It's my poison. It's my medicine. I need it to stop these shakes, these tremors, these leaps of vomit up the back of my throat. A pulsating queue of young people snakes halfway down the block.

I scan the lineup, unzip my duffle bag and pull out the one last thing of value in my life: my laptop. My hands caress its second-skin case, given to me by my sons on my fifty-fourth birthday.

I look down at it for a long moment. This laptop is my life: notes, writings, pictures, training materials for my workshops, patient assessment forms, everything I would want and need to start some semblance of a new life as a therapist in Vancouver.

I swallow hard and shuffle along the line.

"Does anyone want to buy a brand-new laptop?" I hold it out to the people in line. "Does anyone want a new laptop?" I repeat my plea over and over. It gains urgency and volume with each repetition. Each one in turn looks, then looks away, focusing on the flirtatious dance at hand.

"Let me see what you got, old man." A young guy surveys my laptop. He wears a slim-fit white shirt opened to the sternum to reveal freshly waxed, shiny, steroid-enhanced pecs.

"I'll give you twenty bucks." He's rightly assessed he has the upper hand in this negotiation. "That's all I got, dude."

"Twenty bucks? I paid fourteen hundred dollars for it," I stammer.

"Twenty bucks, take it or leave it," he says.

Bastard. In desperation I take it.

My hand shakes as I jerk the twenty-dollar bill from his hand. I walk forty-three paces down the block, into a bar, and order a Rickard's Red. My favourite beer. I down it, and in quick succession order four more. Gone in a matter of forty minutes.

I drop my head onto the bar and the light fades.


I wake up God knows where. I uncurl myself from a fetal position on the only tiny piece of dry concrete in Vancouver, my no fixed address for I think three days now. My splitting head rests on my duffel bag. I fumble for my jacket. It's gone. The beautiful black leather jacket I bought several winters ago when life was good is gone. One by one, pieces of the man I used to be keep disappearing.

A bedraggled fellow with an overflowing shopping cart shuffles past. "Hey, man, you got any extra cash so I can get some breakfast?" He nods at me.

"Beat it," I mutter as I uncoil my stiff and aching body, standing up to get my bearings.

Where the hell am I? 604-298-3250. A surge of clarity rips through my foggy brain like a bullet. 604-298-3250. Dana's sister's phone number. I repeat it over and over as I run around frantically trying to find the payphone I'd used before. 604-298-3250. 604-298-3250. Where's the damn phone? 604-298-3250.

I spot the phone booth beside the liquor store. Inside, I dial the number.

*Pick up. Pick up. Pick up.* Three rings. *Pick up. Pick up. For Christ's sake. Pick —*

"Hello." A tired voice answers the phone,

"It's Mike," I say. "How's Dana? Is she there?"

"Hello, Mike. She won't come out of her room. Only to go to the bathroom or drive to the liquor store to get more to drink."

She calls out, "Dana, it's Mike."

After what seems an eternity that deep, sexy voice, now with an edge of rasp, picks up the phone.

"Oh my God, Mike," Dana says. "Where have you been? You were supposed to be here days ago. I've been phoning everyone in Penticton. Your office manager said you left there on the bus. I thought you were dead. I need you. You have to get here now."

She gives me directions to her sister's place.

I march straight up Main Street to the closest SkyTrain station. The SkyTrain is Vancouver's wondrous aboveground driverless train. No one takes your ticket; it's an honour system. You just buy it and walk on. Tonight, I have no ticket and no honour.

I squish my sodden body and duffle bag into a seat. The train is warm and dry. Everyone reads quietly, texts or just stares into space. In a mere thirteen minutes I will arrive at Metrotown Station.

That gives me thirteen minutes to take stock. Getting on that Greyhound, I abandoned my practice; turned my back on the few loyal clients who still believed in me. I haven't been to my office since the bender began at Todd's little house. I wonder if I even have an office anymore.

At 9:47 a.m., the automatic doors slide open and I step off the train. It's still pouring outside.

It's a short walk past the sixties-era mall, home of the closest liquor store to Dana's mother's home, into post-

WWII suburbia. Tired, I trudge past row upon row of the same Italian-style, stucco-covered bungalow. I tap on the door of 4357 Portland Drive with some trepidation, not sure of what will happen next. I can't wait to see Dana — that pretty red hair, loose strands falling over her cheeks and neck. I can't wait to lose myself in those huge, piercing blue eyes. My stunningly beautiful drinking buddy.

The rust-red door opens and some other woman appears, dressed in grimy white sweat pants and an equally grimy pink terry robe, dirty lifeless hair hurriedly trussed up in pins.

"Well, who the hell is this?" I laugh.

Dana grabs my arm and shoves me into a bedroom immediately to the right of the front entrance. I stare into her dull eyes. Where is my Dana?

"Quick," she whispers. "Get in here."

I smell vodka: Smirnoff. The bottle shimmers mirage-like on the nightstand, the usual blessed forty-pounder and a two-litre bottle of Fresca alongside, with a half-empty glass and ice.

First things first — I reach for the uncapped bottle and take two quick swigs. Brief pause. Breath. Then a third big gulp. Ahhhhhhh. The familiar warmth spreads from my core out to my freezing extremities. The anxiety that buzzed through my entire body and mind mutes. The craving satiated, I focus on Dana.

Dana. How could someone change so dramatically in one week?

"You look terrible. You must have lost ten pounds!" I estimate.

"You don't look so great yourself, Mr. Pond," Dana pulls at her hair. "Where have you been? I've missed you so much. I thought you were dead."

"Downtown Eastside Vancouver." I sit on the edge of the bed.

"What did you do for money?" she asks.

"I'm pathetic at panhandling. I sold my laptop for twenty bucks." The memory of it kicks at my gut.

"Oh my gawd, Mike, not your laptop." Dana shakes her head. She changes gears. "We've got to get out of here." Our eyes lock in longing. "We need to be alone." All at once, Dana dives into her clothes, throws toiletries into an overnight bag, gulps down her drink and calls a cab.

Doris, Dana's sister, hides in her bedroom behind a blaring TV.

The cab arrives and, like the rats we are, we scurry out. Booze has brought us to life. The drunken electric energy between us crackles once again.

"Take us to Metrotown Mall," Dana barks to the driver.

We arrive at the mall and Dana darts into the TD bank. Within minutes she strides out through the pouring rain straight to the government liquor store a few doors down. In a heartbeat she's back in the cab with a brown paper bag full of clinking bottles.

"Take us to the Burnaby Motel." Dana hugs the bag in her lap.

I inspect the contents of the bag and share my approval. "Good work, babe. You're the best." I pull out a vodka cooler, twist the cap off and drain it.

We arrive at the motel and hole up, just like Bonnie and Clyde again. When it occurs to us, we order in: pizza, Chinese food, Thai. More importantly, when our supply runs out, I stagger to the nearest beer and wine store. Dana's phone rings constantly.

Her sister. Her work.

Time and reality suspend. Nothing stops the bender until the money runs out a week later. Dana contacts her friend Vicki, who spends winters in Greece. Vicki agrees to let us stay in her house. We shell out our last few dollars for a taxi. Dana races to the spot where the key is hidden.

"I can't find the fucking key!" Dana's voice rises with panic. "There's no fucking key here!"

It's getting cold and dark. I try to jimmy every window. No go. This place is break-and-enter-proof. Now I'm thinking like a criminal. I find a heavy eight-foot steel pipe at the side of the house. With a long run-up and full force, I ram the door over and over again, taking the occasional break to replenish my drink.

Finally, weakened by successful battering rams, the wooden door gives way and pulls from the frame. We are in. Only one thing matters now: where is the damn liquor cabinet?

We lay waste to Vicki's house. We devour every cracker, every box of cereal, every can of tuna. In five days, we consume literally everything in the house.

Now we both know we're in trouble. We have no money. No booze. No food. Dreaded withdrawal, waiting patiently in the wings, pounces. And so the agony begins again.

Sobriety slinks in, slow and painful.

"Dana, I need to go to the hospital," I say. "This is going to be a bad one."

"I'm not going," she replies.

# 7

# I DON'T WANT TO
# GO TO REHAB

I've been through enough detox to know what comes next. Intolerable vomiting, shakes, fevers, chills, blinding headaches. Every noise magnified ten thousand times. Even the softest touch is too much. And that's if I get off easy.

My first stint in treatment was at Pine-Winds Recovery and Treatment Centre in the Okanagan in November 2005. Taylor and a couple of guys from AA ambushed me. I stayed at Pine-Winds just long enough to detox and then I left. April 2006, a few months later, back to Pine-Winds. Fastforward a few more months and I'm in the back of our Honda Odyssey family van gagging and heaving, yet again in the throes of detox. In the front, Rhonda drove as our family doctor glanced over the seat, his face furrowed with worry. We sped to Kelowna, about an hour's drive away, where Rhonda and my doctor intended to admit me to the psych ward. He wanted to save me, a fellow health care professional, the embarrassment of being hospitalized for alcoholism in my own hometown. All I could think about in the back of that van was my practice. What would become of my practice?

My doctor wanted me certified. I was too sick, too agitated, too distracted to fight him.

As I clung to the edge of the car seat, Rhonda — beyond exasperated, tears in her voice — kept asking the question that I'm still not sure I can answer: "Why would anybody do this to themselves?" She blinked away tears as she drove. "Michael, you have a very serious problem. You are destroying everything you care about. Why? Why? Can't you see what you are doing to all of us?"

She broke down and sobbed until I heard a big long sigh. Then silence.

Why would anyone in their right mind do this to themselves? I'm not in my right mind. I lost it long ago, probably when I was twelve and my brother, Roger, was eleven and we bought a kit to make root beer. We'd heard that if we added yeast, it would get really fizzy. If not capped properly, it would also ferment. We spent half that summer drunk on a bad batch of root beer. Roger and I continued to drink through our adolescence and young adulthood. Most times the booze would be mixed with pot and hash. Acid trips were commonplace. I somehow managed to retain some semblance of control. Roger, on the other hand, would regularly drink himself into oblivion. Every time, I would pack him home from the party, sneak him into the house and plop him in his bed to sleep it off.

I remember when he was thirteen, his friend Don Sutter called me over to their house. Roger had drunk so much of a Texas mickey of cognac and grape Kool-Aid, he'd passed out in a puddle of purple puke. I hoisted him on my shoulder to my car and drove him to the CFB Shilo hospital. He had alcohol poisoning. Then I went home, got my mother and took her to the hospital. When Mum saw Rog unconscious on that hospital bed with a gastric tube in his mouth, she fainted. The nurse had to catch her.

The doctor said, "Get her out of here."

After that, Dad CB'd Roger for a month — confined him to barracks. The only time he was allowed out of his room was to go to the bathroom and school. I remember listening to him cry alone in his room. We weren't allowed to talk to him. My sisters would take him his meals. When Dad wasn't around, we'd sneak him in cookies and powdered milk.

Rog was the family clown. When Dad was hungover and Mum was pissed off, Rog diffused the tension with his jokes. We would laugh so hard at the table, our milk would spew out of our noses. His impressions of all the kids and their parents on the base broke everybody up. He would draw caricatures of everyone he met and then imitate their voices and mannerisms. My aunt Shirley called him Rich Little.

To our great surprise, we both graduated from high school. In our late teens, we both moved out west and began working in psychiatric nursing at the mental institution in Ponoka, Alberta. Our drinking ramped up; Roger's went into overdrive. He drank daily. He smoked pot, hash and banana peels. He took acid, mushrooms and mescaline. He swigged bottles of Benadryl cough syrup. He stole a prescription pad out of a doctor's office and forged prescriptions for Valium, phenobarbital and Demerol. He ended up in jail on fraud charges but escaped a severe sentence when his appendix ruptured. He almost died. One night he took a fistful of the antipsychotic haloperidol. The side effects were so severe, his arms contorted to his sides, his tongue protruded two inches from his mouth, and his body jerked so badly that he couldn't stand. I had to take him to the hospital. I thought he was going to die.

Roger's over-the-top alcoholism allowed me to let myself off the hook. "I'm not like him," I told myself. "I don't have a problem."

I'm exactly like him. He's lost everything already. I'm just a little bit behind.

The doctor, Rhonda and I travelled the rest of the road to Kelowna in stony silence. I stayed one night in the psych ward. Had to get back to my practice.

"No, you don't." Rhonda revealed yet another rehab plan. "Everyone has chipped in to pay for you to attend out of province treatment. Your mum, step-mum, Loretta and Danette all gave me money. You are going to the Claresholm Centre in Alberta." A few hours later I found myself white-knuckling as my plane pitched and rolled its descent through a blanket of heavy wet snow into Calgary, where my mum would pick me up and drive the hour to the treatment centre.

It was a month before Christmas, and my aged mother and stepfather had braved a vicious snowstorm to pick me up and ferry me to treatment. Mum's mouth grimly set, she peered out the windshield as she navigated the treacherous highway. She slowed down to a crawl each time she passed someone spun out in the ditch, enraging all the impatient commuters who aggressively swerved out and passed her. The airline had lost my luggage, so on the way, she pulled in to the snow-packed parking lot of the Deerfoot Mall. We pushed with purpose through the frenzied crowds to Winners for necessities like underwear, deodorant and some T-shirts. I remember Mum pulling out her wallet. Then an odd feel of disconnect. Then nothing.

I came to on the floor of the store. I was on my side in the recovery position, so I wouldn't aspirate. Around me, a circle of winter boots pushed collectively back.

"Give him some air." A gruff, burly ambulance attendant crouched at my side and shone a bright light directly in my eye. Checking my pupil dilation, I surmised. I conducted my own clinical assessment and my heart sank. I'd had a seizure.

It happens after a heavy bender, usually within the initial twelve to forty-eight hours of withdrawal. When alcohol is abruptly withdrawn, the brain kindles, overfires. It doesn't know what to do with itself. Seizures signal end-stage alcoholism. I'd drunk so much booze for so long, my brain could no longer function without it. I needed to keep drinking to prevent seizures. But the very act of drinking was hastening my own death. Addiction is the ultimate paradox.

As I was loaded into the ambulance, I spied my mum, looking small and frail and weary and worried. She had relied on me so much growing up — "Watch your brother and sisters while I go to the store." "Can you get the kids bathed and put them to bed? I have to go to the Al-Anon meeting." My little chest would puff out with pride. I was the man in the family she could rely on. It sure as hell wasn't Dad. Now she was at a stage in life when her burdens should be lightened. What had I done to her? Why couldn't I stop?

Tears welled at the corner of my eyes as the attendants collapsed my gurney and pushed it into the back of the ambulance. At the hospital, I disappeared in the pre-Christmas crush of holiday flu sufferers, just one of dozens way down at the bottom of the triaged list. I waited hours before the attending physician saw me, prescribed Ativan to diminish the chance of another seizure and kept me overnight just in case. He was blunt.

"Mr. Pond, I don't know how to say this in a way you'll listen. Another seizure could kill you. You must stop drinking."

Five o'clock in the morning, Mum was back at the hospital, and in the cold, dark crackling dawn we drove to Claresholm, where I stayed for three weeks.

I was back hard at the bottle within a month. More recriminations and fights between Rhonda and me as the beautiful life we created splintered and shattered. She

43

couldn't keep our masterfully renovated home. The practice wasn't bringing in any money. I saw the clients who would pay me cash, so I could go out and drink right away. Our bills mounted. Lines of credit extended and snapped. Creditors came around, and my boys disappeared into their friends' homes, their girlfriends' lives — anything to escape the insanity of their father's self-destruction.

January 2008: More detox followed by ever harder binges. I no longer slept. I lay in the shelter night after night crushed by mounting anxiety, depression and fear.

My office manager was out to get me.

So was Rhonda — she wanted to ruin me.

I knew that the shelter worker had picked up the phone and called the police. They were coming to put me in the psych ward.

"You're an asshole."

"You've ruined everything."

"You are going down, my friend."

My head jerked around the room. I could hear the voices, but I couldn't see the people.

For the first time, paranoia had hit. In a brief moment of sanity, the professional in me emerged to make the diagnosis: substance-induced psychotic disorder.

In desperation I called my oldest son.

"Hello, Tay, this is Dad."

Long pause. "Who?"

I repeated, "It's Dad."

"Who? Who? Sorry, I don't have a dad. He left a long time ago."

I wished that call was a delusion. But it was cold, hard reality.

I put the phone down and didn't remember anything else.

I came to in the hospital emergency department in restraints, feeling like my back was going to snap in two.

A *second* seizure.

"What is your name and date of birth?" a voice asked.

"Michael Pond, September 27, 1953," I answered.

"Mr. Pond, you had convulsive status epilepticus. Successive severe alcohol-induced seizures," the doctor told me. "If you don't stop drinking, they will kill you."

I was given the anticonvulsant Dilantin, along with phenobarbital and Ativan to take the edge off the withdrawal symptoms. I walked out of the hospital with an envelope containing two more Ativans. *I have to get back to work. My clients need me.*

Who in their right mind would continue to have me as their therapist? Thank God for crazy people who pay cash, whose good sense deserted them long ago, because they kept me in booze. I would have reported me to my governing bodies if I'd had a shred of good sense left.

And that brings us to today, and to Vicki's empty house full of dead soldiers and the familiar shakes. Fear of actually dying of a third seizure, as the doctors predicted, propels me to action.

Dana phones her sister, who drives me to the Creekside Withdrawal Management Centre in Surrey. I am admitted immediately. I conduct my own clinical assessment.

*Clinical Notes — Mental Status Exam:*

*The patient is a short underweight fifty-five-year-old Caucasian male who appears his stated age. He slumps in the chair and avoids eye contact. His clothes are dirty and he is malodorous (alcohol), unkempt and dishevelled. He is incontinent and smells of urine. The patient is guarded and suspicious. His facial expression is perplexed and tremulous. He has psychomotor agitation — ringing his hands, picking his scalp and constant chewing on the inside of his mouth and lips. His speech is low, hesitant and pressured. Affect is depressed and anxious. He reports his mood as depressed and fearful. His cognitive processes show thought blocking, poor concentration and distractibility. The patient is above average intellect; however, short- and long-term memory are impaired. He is oriented to person and place but not time. Thought Content: The patient reports passive suicidal ideation, but denies intent. He expresses guilt, worthlessness and hopelessness. He obsesses about being homeless and penniless. He shows some insight; however, judgment is impaired. Global Assessment of Functioning: 30/100 — Severe impairment. DSM-IV-TR Diagnosis: Alcohol Dependence, Alcohol Withdrawal — Severe.*

With my seizure history, they think it prudent to admit me to the hospital for one night of observation. I agree. And so begins the medically supervised detox all over again. More phenobarbital and Valium. Dilantin wards off seizures. I lie back, seduced by the smell of sanitized pillows and crisp white sheets. It's going to be okay now. I know I can get through this.

The next day, I score a room adjacent to the nurses' station, so they can observe me closely. I feel safe. The drugs begin to work. The wreck that is my life staggers out of the last spectacular crash as rational thought returns. I need to take stock of the damage. I call Rhonda.

"Rhonda, I'm in detox in Vancouver."

"Mike. You're in detox just so you can stay out of jail." Rhonda's steamed. She hasn't heard from me in weeks. In my absence, she picks up the pieces.

And then she drops the bomb.

"I've reported you to your professional bodies, and so has the superintendent of schools. She had a student in crisis and no one could find you. You are in breach of your contract."

I am stunned.

"Rhonda, I can't believe you did this." I try to keep my voice down. "I'm ruined. The whole community will know about my problem now."

"The whole community knows anyway. Who do you think you're kidding, Mike? You abandoned your practice and your clients." She doesn't hide her bitterness.

"But I don't even remember coming down here. Rhonda, I will come back and fix this."

"No, we're shutting it down. Your landlord is evicting you. The boys and I cleared out your stuff." She hangs up.

My practice shut down. Gone. It's all falling apart now.

I call Brennan, my middle son, the only one still speaking to me.

"Dad, we cleared out your office. It was one of the hardest things I've ever done. Taking down all the pictures and your degrees and stuff. Packing up the books and toys in the waiting room. I remember playing with those toys when I was a little kid. I remember bringing in goldfish for the fish tank. It was really hard. One of the saddest days of my life."

"Brennie, I'm in detox in Vancouver. I'm in a lot of trouble. I'm hoping to get into long-term treatment."

"Dad, I hope so. You've got to get better. You just need to keep doing the next right thing."

Next I call my lawyer in Penticton, Matt Jones.

"Mike, where the hell have you been?" Matt shouts. "You're in serious trouble. You're looking at minimum six months in prison."

"I'm in detox, Matt. This time, it's going to stick." I want to believe it's true.

Back in the spring, when I first contacted him, Matt listened wordlessly, like a priest whose physical presence is muted by the mesh of the confessional booth. I offered up a litany of sins. Driving while impaired, driving while suspended, driving while prohibited. Matt and I had shared mutual clients over the years in Penticton and had come to respect each other's work. I suspect he doesn't respect me much now.

He takes in a deep breath and blows it out.

"Get into long-term treatment as soon as possible and I will push the matter forward a few months. This is not good. Not good at all."

I thank him and hang up, suffused with the belief that this time, this time, I'll stay sober.

I can fix this.

Day 4 of detox at Creekside: food stays down, sleep returns, the shakes diminish. I corral my wild erratic thoughts long enough to make a plan. I can turn this around. A few more days at Creekside Detox and I can transfer over to the Phoenix Centre, the long-term treatment my lawyer orders.

When the staff at Creekside discover my background, they are mystified. A young nurse sits down for coffee with me and asks the question I can't answer. "Michael, how did this happen to you? You're a professional. More than anyone, you know the physiological and psychological impact of what you are doing. Why can't you stop?" she said beseechingly.

Here in Creekside, surrounded by detox experts and medications, I believe I can.

I'm deep in conversation with two other male patients when their gazes slide sideways. They look past me in stark admiration. I turn around to see who's putting on the show.

It's Dana. She's decided to join me in detox, like a heat-seeking missile. Every man in the room follows her every calculated step. She plants a kiss on me and gives me a big hug. My reaction is part pride that this fabulous-looking woman wants to be with me and part fear, because holy shit, Dana and I drunk together can get into a whole pile of trouble. Dana and I sober — well, we've never been sober long enough to know. Cautiously, I welcome her to Creekside.

By day's end, Dana has managed to antagonize most of the nurses on the shift. When I suggest she cool it and let them do their jobs, she lashes out. "They're disrespecting me. They're being unkind to me. They're judging me. They are not showing any compassion or understanding. I can tell they hate me." She glares at the nurses' station, willing one of them to challenge her.

Dana with a few drinks is flirty, quick on the uptake and fast with the punchlines. Dana drunk and detoxing is angry.

She sticks it out for six embattled days, enough to get a personal program to stay sober. She talks to a social worker, commits to a day treatment program, calls her sister to pick her up and she's gone. I'll miss her, but I'm relieved.

The next day, a psych nurse named Glen hands me two pieces of mail, one from the College of Registered Psychiatric Nurses of BC and one from the BC College of Social Workers, my two professional regulatory bodies. With dread, I open both. As I speed-read their contents, my gut grips. I sit down. My hands shake. I've been suspended from practising. I am under investigation for malpractice and competency issues. Rhonda and the superintendent of School District 53 submitted complaints about my alcoholism and its impact on my practice. My hands drop to my sides. All the blood leaves my head.

I look at Glen, defeated.

"I've lost my professional licences. I can't do my work anymore," I stammer.

"You're going to get through this, Mike." Glen pats me on the back. "We will get you into treatment. Not just for legal reasons, but to save your life, for yourself. For your life."

Buoyed by his belief, his support, and with Dana out of the picture, I believe I can do it too.

Glen consults with the doctor on my behalf and sits with me as we establish a treatment plan. I have been accepted at the Phoenix Centre. It's brand-new, one of the top addiction centres in the country, and it's only two doors down. As Greg walks me over, I spy the large icon of the Phoenix etched on the façade — the symbol for resurrection.

I begin to feel some hope. I do want help. I do want to recover.

The facility boasts beautiful rooms, a five-star kitchen and a fully equipped gym in the basement. The south half of the building has thirty-six furnished upscale bachelor suites for men in longer-term transition after the initial three months of specialized treatment. I tour through Phoenix Centre wide-eyed and impressed.

I like this place. I like the feel of it. The clients are laughing and smiling. This time I'll stop drinking. I promise.

I check in.


For five weeks at the Phoenix Centre, all through November and early December, I zealously stick to the program. For the first time in three years, I begin to understand the nature of my addiction. Intensive personal and group counselling confirms what my professional insight already knows: the deck is stacked against me.

It begins with a powerful genetic predisposition. And then, for several hours every day as a therapist, I bore witness to terrible stories of hurt and pain and trauma. As the years added up, I became obsessed with this work, addicted to the enormous satisfaction I gleaned from my ability to bring some peace to my tormented clients. I was also addicted to the status my position bestowed. I wanted my wife and kids to want for nothing. The more I worked, the more stuff we could buy. The more stuff we bought, the more I worked.

The healthy way for clinicians to deal with stress is to find another professional to help deal with what's now called vicarious trauma. I debriefed with booze.

At the Phoenix Centre, I develop my own plan for medical monitoring as I maintain sobriety. I establish my own program, and I intend to submit it to my governing bodies. If I stick to it, I'll get my licences back. With all my good behaviour, I earn privileges.

And that's just about the time Dana phones. The sound of her voice delights me. When she suggests a steak at the Keg, I boomerang between exhilaration and unease. There's an old AA saying: Beneath every skirt is a slip. Misogyny aside, there is an element of truth to that old saw.

I'm excited by the possibility of getting out after five weeks. Dana is gorgeous, and I do miss her. But I know she's off the wagon already. If she kicks them back over the ribeye, will I be able to resist?

She drives up in her sister's truck. I haul myself into the cab, and the care she has taken to look good for me takes my breath away. She leans over to kiss me and I smell vodka. She is already tipsy.

My gut cinches. So what? I can do this.

At the Keg, Dana orders double Caesars. I order cranberry and soda. She marvels at my willpower.

"I'm so proud of you, Mr. Pond," she says, and sips her Caesar. "I'm off the wagon already. How do you do it?"

I do it all through dinner, and even when we retire to a hotel room down the street. Dana downs more Caesars as we snuggle on the bed and watch TV. And still I don't drink. But oh God, I want to.

At 10:45 p.m., I'm like the cork on a bottle of champagne — just a bit more pressure and I'll pop.

I can't stand it anymore. I slip off the bed, slide into my clothes and out the door to the liquor store, where I buy a mickey of vodka. I hide the bottle outside and return to the room. I don't want Dana to know. She is so proud of me. I kiss her goodbye and leave before the two a.m. curfew at the Phoenix Centre descends. I grab my bottle from the bush, take a few swigs and head straight there. Swaggering now with boozy bravado — "strutting like a little bantam rooster" is how my grandmother would cluck-cluck her disapproval — I stride past the front desk to my room and tiptoe past my sleeping roommate, directly into the closet. I close the door behind me.

Greedily, clumsily, I all but rip the cap off and down the vodka in minutes. I creep to the third-floor balcony and toss the empty. It lands in a low bank of soggy rhododendrons. Fooled them again.

I fall back onto my bed into a deep and somewhat guilty sleep.

When I wake the next morning, James, the third-floor counsellor, confronts me, disappointment etched into his face. My roommate was awake the whole time. He reported me while I slept it off.

"Mike, you know the drill," James sighs. "The group will now consider what happens next." He leaves me to sit alone in the dining room and watch the kitchen staff in their white smocks and jaunty chef hats.

I stare out of the floor-to-ceiling windows at the darkening sky. Rain whips across the street, and people puddle jump. My shaking hands wrap around what I'm sure is my

last decent cup of coffee for a while. Five weeks of sobriety —
blown.

I wait while the group conscience decides my fate.
"Group conscience" is an AA term that describes how an
entire meeting can reach a consensus on a particular matter.
In AA, the belief is that the group is guided by the higher
power. At the Phoenix Centre, that belief is grounded in a
sense of fair play. I already know what will happen.

James approaches me, his ponytail bobbing. He speaks in
a soft, melodic tone.

"I've got good news and bad news," he says with an
awkward grin. "The bad news is you have to go, Mike. The
group conscience has made its decision. The good news is we
will hold your bed and you can come back in thirty days if
you stay clean and sober."

Fuck. A sickening heat surges up the side of my neck. A
flush floods my face. I'm an idiot. It's December, and outside
looks more like Edmonton than Vancouver. A freak cold
front has settled over the city. Heavy snowflakes tumble from
the sky.

Where will I go? How will I survive? Who will help me
now?

James shakes my hand. "Good luck, Mike. I hope we see
you again in thirty days."

# 8

# GOOD LUCK, MR. POND

I limp out into the main foyer, where my duffle bag and two pieces of Surrey luggage — green garbage bags — filled with my meagre belongings slump at the feet of two guys, Jim and Ron from the third floor.

"We found you a recovery house in White Rock," says Jim. "We're going to take you there right now."

"Thanks, guys," I say. "But I have to go to the bank to get my money." That's another lie. I no longer have a bank account. All my accounts are frozen. I have about seven bucks in my pocket from Dana.

"We'll stop off at the bank on the way," says Ron.

"It's okay. I need some time to myself to think this through. Meet me in the mall in an hour."

I don't give a shit anymore. I just want a drink. The tremors set in. I vibrate inside and out.

I'll panhandle the balance to buy a mickey of the cheap stuff, a dollar less than Smirnoff. In the wake of protests, I powerwalk eight frantic blocks to the mall.

By now I've perfected my panhandling technique. Cold

and honest efficiency. I look 'em straight in the eye: "Do you have a spare loonie?"

No sob story; no bullshit; no explanation.

"Do you have a spare loonie?"

Every fifth or sixth person hands over a shiny coin. Who knows why? Some assuage guilt. Others bear a haunted expression: There but for the grace of God. The rare one meets my gaze with warmth and genuine concern and wishes me well.

I nod in gratitude and express my thanks.

Within half an hour I emerge triumphantly from the liquor store with a mickey of Alberta Springs clutched in my shaky hand. I slip into a public washroom to reload. I brace the door closed because the sliding metal lock is missing. Men come and go and cough and clear their throats and spit. Taps run, and hand dryers whir. The toilet beside me flushes. I gulp big swigs and choke the first few down between gags and heaves. Within minutes the calm envelops me. The rest of the bottle slides down smooth and easy. Deliciously drunk again.

As I stagger through the mall I hear, "Mike, Mike."

I turn and the mall spins dizzily around me. I see Jim and Ron.

I'm not drunk enough to miss the disconcerted glances they exchange.

"Fuck, man, you're pissed. We knew it," Ron shakes his head.

"Let's go!" Jim says. "We're taking you to White Rock. You are so fucked up." He leads me by the arm out of the mall.

We climb into Ron's truck and head south to White Rock, a small, affluent seaside community about forty-five minutes from downtown Vancouver, right on the British Columbia–Washington state border. I haven't been there in twenty years, since my two older boys were five and three. They raced across the expansive White Rock beach begging, "Find some more baby crabs, Daddy. Do your earrings. That's so funny." Rhonda smiled. She was four months pregnant with our youngest, Jonny. I lifted a large rock from the wet sand and scooped two tiny crabs from a troop that was scurrying for cover. I held one gingerly to each ear and their miniature claws clipped onto my lobes. The boys laughed and screamed.

"Daddy wears earrings. Haha. You're so funny, Daddy. Isn't he funny, Mummy?"

"Oh yes. He is so, so funny," she said with a sardonic grin.

Today the beach is all but obliterated by a wall of thick, pelting snow. The wind wails incessantly; the snow piles two feet deep against pounding grey surf. It's the beginning of the worst winter in sixty-four years. I couldn't be further from that young, exuberant, sober father.

At the recovery house, a woman waits at the door for me.

Jim explains, "She runs this house and a few others in town."

"How are you going to pay?" the well-dressed, middle-aged south Asian woman demands.

"I've applied for social assistance," I say. "I'm still waiting to hear."

"We'll take you to the welfare office tomorrow," Jim assures me.

Jim and Ron dump my duffle bag at the front door.

"You're going to be okay," Ron calls out from the truck as they get back in.

I walk into my bedroom and a young guy lying on the other bed mutters, "She's sleeping with one of the clients here."

This offends my drunk self, which is a crock because who am I to claim the moral high ground? Without a word I pick up my duffle and garbage bags and stagger out the door into the biting cold. Wearing a thin jacket and runners, I wander the streets of White Rock. I don't even have a quarter to make a phone call. What's worse, I have no one to call. I huddle behind a dumpster in the alley behind a row of restaurants. Then I spy the Boathouse — an old family favourite. I stagger in, drawn by the warmth. A young blond hostess greets me with a look like I am a creature from another planet.

"Can I help you, sir?"

"I'm sorry, I have no money for the payphone. Can I use your phone to call a friend?"

"I'm not sure," she squeaks. "I'll have to ask my manager."

As she disappears around the corner, I notice the place is empty. A young fellow wipes and sets tables. He busies himself out of sight. Blood floods into my extremities and my fingers are on fire. Even more painful is the unquenchable urge to drink.

Behold the superbly laid out and highly stocked bar. My lover's gaze lingers on the vodkas, then comes to rest on the Scotch. If I just stretch a bit, I can grab a bottle. But I can't possibly steal a bottle of booze from the Boathouse.

Yes, I can. It would be no different from the dozens of times I strode confidently into the Penticton liquor stores, picked up two bottles of Smirnoff, shot a swift glance around to ensure I was out of sight of security cameras and people — then stuffed one bottle in my pants, walked up to the clerk and paid for the other.

No different from the summer I broke into my accountant's cabin next door and took a bottle of her expensive Snow Queen vodka. Police told her that if she pressed charges, I'd get help. She agreed. The Summerland RCMP charged me with break and enter and theft, my first drinking-related charge. I received a conditional sentence and no record. The only condition was to get treatment and go to AA. And I did ... for a while.

I scan the restaurant. No one in sight. The pretty hostess will be back any minute. I must move fast.

A brief flash of another Mike Pond makes me hesitate: honest contributing citizen, family man, hockey coach, the man I used to be — he wouldn't dream of doing this. But that Mike Pond doesn't live here anymore. That unbearable, beyond-any-logic-and-understanding desire drowns out reason.

I zero in on a bottle of Glenfiddich 12 single-malt Scotch. With surprising deftness, I reach up, seize the trophy and shove it inside my jacket just as the hostess comes around the corner of the bar.

With a look of regret she murmurs, "I'm sorry, sir, the manager says you can't use the phone. Unless you want service, you will have to leave."

I can't wait to get my ass out of there. I duck into the washroom, slither down the stall wall and pull out my precious prize. The first hot swallow hits the wall in the back of my throat. Five deep rapid breaths push it down. A straight arm against the wall of the stall steadies me. My head dips expectantly over the toilet. The next gulp is bigger and easier to keep down. My stomach welcomes it now and the warm, numb glow fills my entire being. Nothing matters anymore except this feeling. Everything else disappears. My kids. Homelessness. Being broke.

I head out into the midday cold and stumble down the isolated boardwalk. The freak winter storm continues to batter the entire lower mainland of British Columbia. The snow-clogged streets lie silent. The wild ocean wind shoves me sideways, making it even more difficult to negotiate an already unsteady search for sanctuary. I take shelter behind a log on the beach. I take another long, full swig of my delicious Scotch friend and snuggle with him close to my chest. I don't feel the chill anymore.


Reluctant eyelids peel open. My body shudders. It's cold again. I fumble unconsciously for the elusive blanket. A metal door clangs and boot steps echo down a concrete hall. The familiar smell of old paint and piss invades my nostrils. I'm in jail again.

The small window shutter slides open.

"It's time to go."

I mutter through a cotton mouth, "Where am I?"

"White Rock RCMP cells. A couple walking their dog on the beach found you behind a log. They thought you were dead. We brought you in. You were half-frozen. I've got to release you."

My jeans are wet. Lovely. I've pissed myself.

"What time is it?" I ask.

"Oh-three-eighteen."

"In the morning?" I blink and look around.

"Yep. You were brought in early last night."

The corporal's key opens the door and he leads me down the concrete hall to the desk. He heaves my duffle bag onto the counter and pecks on his keyboard.

"You have no ID. What's your name?"

"Michael Pond."

"Date of birth?" He types my information into the computer database.

"September 27, 1953."

"You've got quite a record here, Mr. Pond — a lot of alcohol-related charges and convictions." He looks up from his screen. "You could have died out there last night. This is brutal weather. You're lucky those folks found you."

"I have nowhere to go." It's starting to become my mantra.

The corporal slides my duffle bag across the stainless steel counter.

"There's a United Church just around the corner on Pacific Avenue. They have an emergency shelter set up because of the bad weather. They may be able to help you." He gets up out of his chair, keys in hand. "I'll let you out the front door. Good luck, Mr. Pond."

I shoulder my duffle bag and step out into the cold darkness. The crackly air shocks my lungs. I squint at the road sign: Pacific Avenue. To the north, a block and a half away, is the church. Sick and disoriented, I make my way to the back entrance.

A sign on the door reads White Rock Temporary Shelter.

I open the door and the aroma of hot coffee and cocoa beckons.

"Come in, come in. Are you okay?" A young guy, his face flooded with concern, leads me to the church kitchen and hands me a hot chocolate and two Tim Hortons muffins.

In my days as a hockey dad, stomping my feet in frozen arenas, I mindlessly downed cup after cup of Timmy's. Now I savour every precious sip.

"I was just released from the RCMP cells around the corner," I say between sips. "Someone found me on the beach yesterday passed out."

"You can stay here till six thirty," he says, "then we need to clear the church out. You can come back this evening at nine. Crash on one of the mats over there, okay?" The young guy points me toward the mats, then goes to greet another newcomer.

It's a large hall, like an old high school gymnasium, the raised stage bumped and scratched from decades of Christmas pageants and year-end recitals. A Christmas tree stands forlornly at the back of the stage, a nativity scene at its feet. A large, sliding room divider is half open, revealing a circle of wooden collapsing tables with stackable chairs around its perimeter. A single row of mats with blankets line up along the long wall below the windows.

I collapse onto a mat. It's comfortable and warm. Half a dozen snoring bodies lie in a row alongside me. An old white-bearded fellow curled up beside me murmurs, "It's brutal out there, eh? I've been on the streets for eighteen years and I've never seen a winter like this. Thank God for this church, eh? I'm pretty damned sure I woulda froze to death this past week."

"Yeah. It just feels good to have something warm in my stomach." I shut my eyes.

I wake up with the young church guy gently shaking my shoulder.

"It's time to go, sir. I have a voucher here for a breakfast meal at McDonald's."

"But I have nowhere to go." It's a limp protest now.

Nowhere to go. Nowhere to go. I have to say it a few times before it sinks in. Oh my God. I am truly homeless now, just like the decrepit old man being nudged awake beside me. I gaze across at him. Raw fear like I've never before experienced grips my heart and won't let go. No more second-rate motels or hostels. No more couch surfing or sleeping in my truck or crashing in my office. No more home.

"I'm really sorry." The young guy shrugs. "There's an AA meeting here this morning at seven. Why don't you stay for that?"

He points to a middle-aged fellow making carafes of coffee with a Bunn industrial drip machine.

"That guy over there may know someone who can help you."

I've had an on-again, off-again relationship with AA for years now. I hate to go to the meetings because doing so means I have to admit I have a drinking problem. Rhonda, desperate for me to get help, used to drive me to Kelowna, an hour's drive from home, so I could attend a professionals' AA meeting. She'd drop me off, go shopping and come back to get me an hour and a half later.

I never went in. I went shopping, too — at the nearest bar.

Now I have no choice. This AA meeting is the only place I have to go. I walk over to the guy on coffee duty. We shake hands.

"My name's Clifford," he says. "There's a big meeting here every morning. I'll introduce you to some of the guys."

Exhausted, dehydrated, I'm barely aware of time passing by. My head droops loosely on my shoulders, and saliva pools and dribbles from the sides of my mouth as I nod in and out of sleep. Like time lapse on TV, each time I come to, more bodies fill the room. By seven a.m. the hall holds over seventy-five people, mostly men, of all ages.

AA meetings typically begin with the Serenity Prayer: "God grant me the serenity to accept the things I cannot change, courage to change the things I can and the wisdom to know the difference."

"Is anyone coming back?" the chair asks.

AA experience tells me I will be asked to share. I'd prefer to sit in silence with my shame. My hand slides up, sheepish and slow.

"My name's Mike, I'm an alcoholic. I've slipped and slid in and out of AA and sobriety for three years," I say to the packed hall. "I just can't seem to stay sober. I've lost my family, my home, my career, and my self-respect. In the last six months, I've moved from a beautiful and successful life in the Okanagan to living as a down-and-out skid-row bum on the Downtown Eastside. I sold my brand-new laptop for five beers. I've probably been to a half-dozen treatment programs. Drunk tanks, hospitals, detox centres — I know them all. I've had seizure after seizure. I've racked up half a dozen drunk-driving-related charges. Every day, I thank God I never hurt or killed anyone. My kids don't talk to me. I have nothing left." I stop to take a breath.

"And yet, I don't seem to be able to quit. I've even come close to dying. I've been told my ego will kill me. I've been told I need to 'let go and let God.' I've been told I just haven't surrendered yet. Well, where do you sign up for that? I'm surrendering today." I sit back down.

The meeting ends as it started, with the Serenity Prayer. Several guys envelop me in a circle of encouragement, urging me to just stay sober today.

"Just for today, Mike, one day at a time," one guy says, nodding.

"We're from a recovery house just down the road," an older guy says. "Why don't you come with us? Jump in the bus."

Before I leave with them, I seek out a female member of AA and press Dana's phone number into her hands.

"Tell her I'm going to rehab. Tell her I'm going to be okay."

The woman smiles and I manage a shaking half-grin back.

I follow the men to the church parking lot through the still-raging blizzard as daylight finally breaks. A white minibus sits idling. Blue letters along the side spell out the next stage of my life: "The Fresh Start Addiction Recovery Society." Several men huddle behind it sucking cigarettes and diesel exhaust. The bus fills with men of all ages and sizes. I look back at the church, the snowstorm, the smoking men and climb inside the minibus. The black vinyl seat presses ice cold through my thin, piss-damp jeans. I feel a rush of warm air from the dash. I close my eyes, rest my head against the window and fall asleep.

# 9

# THE FRESH START ADDICTION RECOVERY SOCIETY

"Welcome to the handy DART bus of mentally retarded alcoholics." I wake with a start.

A kid no older than my youngest son is bellowing at me from another seat.

"We're a bunch of losers living in a condemned old folks' home." He snickers. "Hey, old man, you're gonna feel right at home. Ha ha, you old fuckin' loser."

"Lenny, sit down and shut the fuck up," yells the driver.

"You shut the fuck up, Monk." Lenny sneers. "You big fat bag of shit."

Monk is a big man in his mid-thirties. He stands six foot three and weighs in at 310 pounds, and that's on a day when he's watching his weight. He keeps his head shaved and holds a second-degree black belt in tae kwon do. For his heft, he moves with the stealth and grace of a cat.

On cue from Monk, a guy in a jean jacket and black Dayton boots springs up, grabs Lenny in a chokehold and drags him back, hard into the rear of the bus. Lenny's arms wave frantically, and within seconds he slumps unconscious into the back seat.

Monk peers into the rear-view mirror.

"Thanks, Brad," Monk nods. "That's one way to shut that mouthy little fucker up."

This is my introduction to life at Fresh Start.

I find out later the kind of guy Monk used to be: a feared drug enforcer who moonlighted as a bouncer in one of the highest-end strip bars in Vancouver. When he was twenty-one, he lost his best friend to a drug- and alcohol-related suicide. He was a wounded raging bull until he quit boozing and partying and found God two years ago.

The seven-minute ride to Fresh Start feels like an eternity. Twenty-five men crammed in, swearing and yelling. My head aches and my stomach growls. The bus rolls to a stop in a snowy gravel driveway. We pile out and trudge through knee-deep heavy snow, pounding a path to the back door.

The Fresh Start Recovery House sits on a large corner lot overlooking Semiahmoo Bay. It hides behind a six-foot brown wooden fence and massive Douglas fir trees. The white 1960s single-storey main building sags under the weight of too many sad-sack stories. Off the front entrance sits a two-storey section — an add-on that houses staff apartments. A large yard dominates one side and the back. In the back beside a shed is a rusty metal swing set.

As we cram inside, the floors smear with slushy mud. Overheated, mouldy and musty, the air stinks of stale cigarettes. Several men crowd a small foyer, drinking coffee and eating toast.

As I soon learn, though it's a relatively short drive from South Surrey, Fresh Start might as well be a million miles from the safety, security and medical supervision of the Phoenix Centre.

A young short stocky guy in his early thirties extends

a large, muscular arm to me. "Welcome to Fresh Start." He shakes my hand. "They call me Tom 'Guns.' I got here 'bout three months ago. You don't look so good."

"My name's Mike, and yeah, it's going to get worse."

"Detoxin', eh? Hey, man, you look really familiar. Have I met you before? Surrey? Newton? No, I know. Kelowna!" Tom scrutinizes my face.

"I'm from the Okanagan." I shrug. "Maybe from there."

We stare at each other as he hands me a coffee. My foggy brain flips through thousands of case files until I find him: "Tom 'Guns.'"

"I worked with you in juvie," I tell him. "You were just a kid." I first met Tom as an adolescent at the Youth Detention Centre in the early nineties. He earned the nickname from his juvenile delinquent peers, who stood in awe of his massive biceps.

"Yeah, I know. I've been fucked up a long time." Tom laughs and shakes his head in disbelief. "Holy shit, man."

My presence here in front of him in this rundown recovery home is out of time and out of place.

"How did you end up in this hole?" Tom looks shocked. "You're a professional shrink. You helped me a lot back then."

"Looks like I could have done a better job, eh, Tom?" I sip my coffee. "On you and myself."

"Yeah, man." Tom laughs humourlessly. "This building should be condemned. Other than on the streets, this is as bad as it gets. Actually, sometimes I'd rather be on the streets." He surveys my skinny body.

"You should have something to eat," he says.

"I'm hungry but I can't eat. I'd puke it right back up."

Tom nods. He knows the detox drill.

"Eli will put you on the couch of willingness," he says, with a dark note in his voice. "Do you know what that is?"

I take a guess. "Where the new guy bunks out so the staff can determine how willing he is to get clean and sober? Like a probationary period?"

"Yep, that's right. Let me show you around. Then go lie down. You look like shit." Tom takes me on a tour. The halls are narrow and dark, the rooms small. Single-sized rooms are crammed with two, sometimes three beds. Dust layers upon grime upon dirt. I stop at a closet-sized bathroom to relieve myself. Even for a guy straight off the streets, the filth disgusts me. I postpone my pee and rejoin Tom's tour.

"Who's Eli?" I ask Tom.

"Eli is the guy who founded Fresh Start. He's ex-army. Sobered up when he was fifty and opened this place. His way of giving back, I guess. He's a diehard AA old-timer. Runs this place like a drill sergeant. Don't get on his bad side." Tom shoots me a look of warning.

We walk into a small lounge with glass doors leading out to a patio and generous garden area. Massive cedar trees, heavy with fresh snow, stand sentry over the sprawling lot. With his bulging arm, Tom gestures to two old sofas in the lounge.

"Those are the couches of willingness. You'll be sleeping on that one. There's another one outside in the smoke pit. Too cold out there right now. But when the weather's good, it's the best couch. I know. I've been on them all."

Several men sit smoking on sixties-era living-room furniture in an area off the kitchen. Butts fill an ancient standing glass ashtray.

"Practically everything here has been scrounged or donated," Tom explains. "We get a lot of the food from the local grocery stores and Cobs bakery. It's expired and just gets thrown out."

I'm starved but my stomach recoils at the thought of food, and it shows on my face.

"Lie down and rest, Mike," Tom says. "Maybe you'll feel like eating in a bit. I'll get you some sheets and blankets."

I collapse on the vacant couch. My butt sinks deep into the worn brown corduroy cushion. The springs complain with a rusty whine. I rest my head on the round arm and get a whiff of the pillow. I bolt upright. It stinks of booze-tinged sweat, vomit and urine. Tom returns with an armful of linen, blankets and a stained pillow. "The couch is a test of your willingness, Mike, your willingness to surrender. Your willingness to do what it takes to get sober. Eli and Josh will be watching you. If you don't follow the program, they'll kick you out. You could be here a couple of days. You could be here a couple of months. You could be out on your ass."

I make up my couch of willingness as men meander in and out of the patio doors and down the dim hallway to their respective rooms. The couch is situated in the busiest access route in the house. Men come and go continually from outside, the dining room and the main living area. There will be no peace, no quiet and absolutely no privacy.

"You gotta surrender, buddy. Or you're gonna die. Guaranteed," growls a raspy-voiced old guy shovelling a bowl of Corn Flakes into his three-toothed mouth. He drags his shirtsleeve across his face to wipe a dribble of sugary milk off his unshaven chin. "Eli will kick your ass outta here if you don't. You'll be back on the streets suckin' cock to make ends meet. Hahaha!"

I shudder to think what my ex-wife Rhonda would think of how the guys talk here. But that's the way they talk in my new world. We, the bottom feeders. If there was any other way to sober up, we've exhausted it. Failed at it. The desperately poor, mentally ill alcoholics and addicts, the brain-injured and more upscale rehab rejects like me all rub shoulders with genuine psychopaths, convicted killers, gangsters and drug dealers who prefer to serve a conditional sentence here than in prison. I conduct another clinical assessment.

*Clinical Notes — Mental Status Exam:*

*Appearance and Behaviour: Patient is a short Caucasian male in his mid-fifties with grey hair. Clothing dirty. Incontinent and smells of urine. Avoids eye contact.*

*Speech: Rapid and disjointed.*

*Mood and Affect: Affect is anxious and depressed. Reports depression and feelings of hopelessness.*

*Thought Content and Process: Obsessive thoughts to obtain alcohol. Belief that life is not worth living anymore. Passive suicidal ideation. Paranoid ideation with psychotic features.*

*Cognition: Time disorientation. Poor concentration. Short-term memory deficit.*

*Insight and Judgment: Insight fair, judgment poor. Minimizes seriousness of illness.*

*Global Assessment of Functioning: 40/100 — Major Impairment.*

*Diagnosis: Alcohol Dependence and Withdrawal. Major Depressive Episode. Anxiety Disorder NOS.*

A lot of guys here suffer from what mental health professionals call "concurrent disorders." They are bipolar disorder and alcoholic, or crackhead schizophrenics. They probably began drinking or taking illegal drugs in their teens, as some desperate kind of self-medication. They won't kick their habit until their mental condition is under control. And that will never happen at Fresh Start. Because the cruel irony here is that just when these guys need medication most, it's forbidden. Fresh Start only accepts clients who are not on any medication. No selective serotonin reuptake inhibitors, no lithium, no trazodone. Which makes it damn near impossible to truly recover in this recovery house.

But for now, it's warm and dry. Since I spent half of last night passed out on White Rock Beach, I'm still chilled to the core. It feels good just to sleep on something soft. It feels good, but I am afraid. What if I can't stay here? What if this man Eli kicks me out?

A chorus of laughter bounces through the common area as I close my eyes to shut out the commotion. Memories of our beautiful home on Lake Okanagan flood in. The boat bow slices open the sandy brown and green mountains reflected on the glass-topped water. The hot sunny wind presses my Ray-Bans against my suntanned face. I'm young and vigorous, with a cold bottle of Corona clasped in my left hand. Bruce Springsteen rocks through the Harman Kardon speakers. I gaze into the oversized rear-view mirror as Taylor cuts across the wake and launches fifteen feet into the dry desert air.

"Do a three-sixty, Tay!" Jonny whoops.

"No, Taylor! Do a Raley with a grab!" Brennan counters.

Life doesn't get any better. We live in paradise.

"Hey, buddy! Eli wants to talk to you."

I open my eyes. Two faces peer down at me.

"I'm Josh, the manager. Me and Eli wanna talk to you."

This is my first introduction to the power duo in charge of Fresh Start.

The taller guy in his late sixties, with the greying red close-cropped hair, is Eli. The boss. He's got a big nose and beady eyes. Next to him stands Josh the house manager. He's squat, trucker-like, mid-fifties and all business.

The three of us go around the corner to a tiny, cluttered office off the dining area, which looks like an old nursing-station medication room. On the wall hangs a framed collage of snapshots of maybe a hundred men. A significant number of them are randomly circled with a black fine-point marker.

"Those guys?" Eli says. "They're dead now. OD'd, suicided, murdered. That's what happens to alcoholics who don't surrender." Eli talks like he's got a mouth full of marbles.

He sits at the small desk facing the window that overlooks the tiny dining room. He speaks in abrupt, sharp-muttered utterances. Worships the Big Book of AA — the only way to recovery. He's convinced.

"Josh tells me you have quite a story. Well-educated professional, eh? Psychotherapist. This disease takes no prisoners," he says.

To Eli I'm just another down-and-outer. No status here. It dawns on me: I *am* just another down-and-outer.

"It costs $550 a month for the program here," Eli explains. "That covers everything. How are you going to pay, guy?"

"I'm broke. I don't qualify for social assistance. They say I have assets. I've been out of my home in Penticton for a couple of years."

"That's what happens," Eli nods. "Alcoholism is the great subtractor. You lose everything, then jails, institutions and death. Josh will take you in to Social Services. If you can't get welfare, you're going to have to find work. We're not a charity."

"I'm going to get my wife to send my degrees and CV

down. I hope I can get work psych nursing or a social work position somewhere."

Eli stares at me like I'm not getting it.

"Hey, guy, your degrees don't get you sober. Are you ready to surrender yet? Start reading the Big Book, and when you're done detoxing, start working on your steps. No, start working on Step 1 right now: Admit you're powerless over alcohol — your life's become unmanageable."

I wobble on shaking legs. The harsh reality of how far I've fallen has just sunk in. As a psychotherapist, I'd always been vaguely aware of the sliding scale of treatment options for addiction. If you've got money or are lucky enough to hold a job in a profession protected by a powerful union, or you're a lawyer in a genteel firm, you'll be sent off to a high-end treatment centre for as long as it takes, followed by intense follow-up care in the community. The back pages of a magazine to which I subscribed, *Psychology Today*, are full of ads for such places. Some charge $45,000 for one month.

Stays in government-licensed and -funded treatment centres, like the Phoenix, are often paid for by the Department of Mental Health and Addictions. If you get kicked out of facilities like these, as I did, you often disappear into a netherworld of unlicensed, unregulated recovery homes. There are hundreds in British Columbia alone. To open one up, all you have to do is incorporate a non-profit society. Clients are all on welfare and hand over their cheques for room and board and what passes for treatment. I suppose there are some recovery homes that provide genuine, medically informed treatment. I just haven't been in one. In my experience, treatment is most often a ride to the closest AA meeting.

I shuffle out of the office and collapse onto the corduroy couch of willingness. My body trembles uncontrollably. Hot chocolate and bran muffin spew into the plastic bucket Tom

"Guns" thoughtfully left at the side of the couch for me. I feel haunted by the black-circled faces of the men who never made it.

I grasp at snippets of sleep, broken by incessant arguing and put-downs throughout the day and by head-ringing snoring at night. Each morning at six the men gather in the dining area and read from the Big Book.

AA's unique blend of compassion and discipline has worked for millions. Eli's militaristic approach delivers cold discipline with almost cultish fervour. But I'm not convinced Eli's version will work for me. Upon each man's arrival, Eli directs him to "personalize" his copy of the Big Book.

"Every place you see a 'we' or 'us,' scratch it out and put 'me' and 'I.' Take full fucking responsibility for yourself and the damage you've done! The Big Book says you're selfish, self-centred and self-seeking. That is the root of your troubles."

Well, to Mike Pond the professional therapist, it's not that simple, and it's clear I need to set the record straight.

"I tend to lean toward a more eclectic interdisciplinary approach," I say. "Using appropriate medication and an integrative blend of different models, like cognitive behavioural therapy, motivational interviewing, family therapy, SMART Recovery and relapse prevention. Evidence-based holistic, multifaceted treatment. Along with being a disease, alcoholism is a systemic problem." I pride myself upon being able to remember all the current buzzwords about addiction treatment.

All the men's eyes turn my way, then dart back to Eli.

He glares at me, then erupts.

"What the fuck do you know about recovery! Look where your fuckin' SMART Recovery got you. You're in a condemned old folks' home, for fuck's sake. You've lost everything. Your selfishness is going to kill you! God makes that possible. Follow the program, guy, or get the fuck out!"

His words sting like a slap. He is right. I am at the bottom of the bottom of the bottom. There will be no holistic approach here, only Eli's. I see what happens to guys who won't follow the program Eli's way. Trent, a heroin addict from a well-to-do family, arrived here after a failed stint at the Orchard, a high-end treatment centre on Bowen Island, just off the coast of Vancouver. He's relapsed multiple times. His grandmother just died, he's depressed and he won't come out of his room. He won't participate, won't attend Eli's program, so he's out on his ass.

"Alcoholics are wilful and ego-driven. Self-will run riot," says Eli. I know that part's true. I also know that it would be challenging not to be hardened, dealing with alcoholics and addicts day in, day out for years. We lie and cheat and steal and scam, and our word, as long as we are using, is worth nothing. Maybe Eli operates like a drill sergeant because it's the only way to survive dealing with us. In a place like this, perhaps a more compassionate guy would be chewed up and spit out in a day.

Eli's unshakable belief in his way or the highway befuddles some of the guys. He forces everyone to admit he's an alcoholic, which is a mind-bender to the guys who are dope fiends. After the early-morning AA meeting, a fellow member of the house tells me Eli forced him to say he was an alcoholic.

"I'm not an alcoholic," he says. "I don't even like booze. I'm a crackhead, and I love crack. I don't understand how admitting I'm an alcoholic will help me kick crack." He shakes his head.

Thank God I'm a plain-and-simple alcoholic. I love booze. I am anxious to stay on Eli's good side, so I get with his program. I start to memorize the Big Book.

On my seventh day at Fresh Start, I take my first shower. Brown and yellow scum coats the shower stall. Slime and pubic hairs cover the toilet. And then I laugh to myself. There is some irony in a guy who hasn't showered in seven days protesting the cleanliness of the shower stall.

I close my eyes, take a deep breath and step in.

The hot water cascades over my face. The filth fades and I stand in the walk-in white marble shower of our newly renovated home on the lake. My morning routine before I head to the office unfolds: a steamy americano on the deck with the morning paper; I scan Skaha Beach as the early-morning strollers walk their dogs; birds chirp and a golden retriever scatters a gaggle of Canada geese off the sand; they fly low about forty feet and skim along the water off shore to taunt the barking dog, just out of reach—

"Get out of the shower, dude." Someone pounds on the door. "You're using up all the hot water."

I towel dry, pull on my filthy donated jeans and grimy shirt and smile in spite of myself. I've worn the same pair of underwear for a week. My mother would be ashamed.

From this day on, I clean the bathroom in my wing, every day.

Later that day, Josh speed-waddles toward me in the dining room.

"Let's go. We're going to Social Services. You gotta apply for welfare."

At the Surrey Ministry for Housing and Social Development office, the lineup trails out the door and halfway around the block. People smoke and cough and curse the brutal weather and curse the government and stomp and sway in the frosty air.

I've never collected welfare or unemployment insurance in my life. Started working when I was fourteen. I retreat deep into myself, physically curling inward, partly in response to the cold, partly to hide my shame. I hope no one I know drives by.

After two hours inching forward in the frigid lineup, I meet a social worker in her mid-twenties. Her young brow furrows, perplexed.

"Your file from the Phoenix Centre indicates you have significant assets and property in Penticton." She looks me right in the eye. "You don't qualify for financial assistance."

I must. Without money to pay Eli, I'm homeless. I meet her stare.

"I'm an alcoholic who has lost pretty well everything. What's left, I can't access. I am over ninety thousand dollars in debt. I plan to sign the house and everything over to my ex-wife to make amends for all the damage I've done to my family."

"You're too mentally ill right now to make that kind of decision," the social worker says. "You need to see a psychiatrist. You need legal advice as well."

"I'm in treatment. I'm a professional therapist. I'm also a psych nurse. I'm going to appeal to my professional associations to have my licence to practise reinstated. I plan to get work at a local hospital. I'll take any nursing or social work job I can get." Desperation creeps into my voice.

The social worker takes in the whole sorry sight of me. And she relents.

"Wait a minute, Mr. Pond. I'm going to talk to my supervisor."

A minute becomes twenty minutes. I count every one on the large institutional clock as I wait alone in her office. I imagine the conversation they're having about me. I wouldn't believe me either. She finally returns. And she's smiling.

"I've talked to my supervisor. We will grant you six months of social assistance under the hardship clause. During that time you will be required to retain a lawyer,

settle your separation agreement and find work. Your assistance will then be cut off. Good luck, Mr. Pond."

How many times now have I heard that — "Good luck,
Mr. Pond"? Police, doctors, nurses, lawyers, social workers,
all seem invested in me getting my shit together.

My monthly welfare check is $610. Fresh Start takes $550
for room and board. That leaves $60 a month for everything
else. I used to spend that on lunch and a glass of Chardonnay.

Back at the house, Tom "Guns" conspiratorially gestures
me his way.

"Hey, Mike," he whispers. "A woman has been calling all
day for you on the house phone. She sounds loaded."

10

# A FRESH START
# CHRISTMAS

Dana!

"That's my girlfriend, Dana," I burst out. Dana, my last connection to the life I used to have.

"Man, she's got a hot voice." Tom grins. "Call her on my cell if you want. Don't let anyone see, though. You'll get kicked outta here if Eli finds out you're on the phone, especially with a woman. And a drunk bitch at that."

I duck around the back of the building behind a large cedar tree.

"Hi, Dana," I whisper. My voice drips with longing. The words catch in my throat.

"One of the guys at the Phoenix Centre told me where you were. I miss you, Mr. Pond. I need you." Her voice is deep and husky. I crave her. I also crave a drink. The two are becoming indistinguishable.

"It's Christmas in a couple of days," says Dana. "I will come and get you from that hellhole. You don't belong with all those crackheads and criminals. You're a professional, Mr. Pond."

I am a professional — a professional drunk.

"Okay," I say. "Call Tom on this number when you're ten minutes away."

"I'll be there, Mr. Pond. I can't wait to see you. We'll get a hotel."

Dread and exhilaration duke it out in my head. The thought of Dana's long silky legs, her dancing mischievous eyes, her bed-tousled red hair makes me want her here, right now. But a few days of sobriety reward me with fresh insight: the two of us together are a train wreck.

Then, like an apparition, Monk's huge body glides up in the snow.

I slam Tom's phone shut.

"Pond," Monk says. "You're not supposed to be on a phone. Two weeks, then you get privileges. Get your shit. You're off the couch. You're gonna bunk with Dangerous Doug."

In my new room, Dangerous Doug lies on his bed reading a paperback.

"I hate this fuckin place and all the fuckheads in it," Doug says into his book. "I'd kill every one of them if I got the chance. Get outta here as soon as you can, buddy."

Twenty-five years of hard drinking cost Dangerous Doug everything. He's a mean drunk. He's relapsed twice in the last three months and fought both times with a couple of the young men in Fresh Start, who tease him. I've drawn the short straw. Only one sleep, though, until I see Dana.

After ten days on the couch of willingness, I should be thankful for my real bed. But as night falls and Dangerous Doug slips into fitful sleep interrupted by huge snoring snorts, I am not thankful at all.

I lie awake and obsess about whether seeing Dana is a good idea. How can seeing Dana ever be a good idea? The fact I actually have this debate with myself is testament to how much my judgment is impaired.

Ever since my last bender during the blizzard, I've been sober. Just over a week. I survived yet another detox. But Dana is temptation itself. I can't stop thinking about her. I miss her. I can't admit to anyone, even to myself, just how lonely I have become.

I look out the window. The snow shimmers in the soft moonlight. Clouds scud past the moon and reveal a twinkly starlit sky. In the claustrophobic misery of Fresh Start, it's easy to forget there's still a wide-open beautiful world beyond the six-foot fence. I gaze out and watch the stars fade, replaced by the grey slate dawn. The clouds look heavy again. More snow.

I attend the mandatory AA meeting that morning. I begin the Serenity Prayer. "God grant me the ... yeah yeah yeah blah blah blah ... and the wisdom to know the difference."

I struggle more and more with Eli's version of AA. Real AA embodies love and tolerance and acceptance and one day at a time. At Fresh Start, I am surrounded by intolerance, judgment and shame. The dissonance of the hypocrisy dilutes the power of the program. Yet it works for some of the guys. Men credit Fresh Start with saving their lives. And I desperately need the support of a sponsor.

An AA sponsor is a member with significant sobriety, experience and knowledge in the program to guide and support a co-member. It's strongly suggested that you have a sponsor — another level of accountability and commitment to the program.

After the meeting I mechanically eat several pieces of Cobs-donated white-bread toast and drink coffee after coffee. The artificial whitener leaves a vague petrochemical taste in my mouth.

My internal debate about seeing Dana escalates. Am I still searching for excuses to fail? Clearly, I'm not quite ready to surrender yet.

I play crib. It's a popular game in recovery and treatment centres. It kills time and conversation. The schoolhouse clock above the fireplace reads 9:13 a.m.

Brad deals the usual six cards each. It's his crib.

"There you go, Professor Pond. Read 'em and weep."

I survey my hand. Two fives. Two Jacks. A six of spades and an eight of hearts. Nice! I flick the six and eight to Brad. He slaps two cards face down on top of mine.

"You're gonna get skunked, Doctor Pond. I just dumped a seven and an eight in my crib." I cut the deck and Brad flips over a seven of clubs and yelps, "Yes! Come to Papa. You lead, sucker." I fight back the urge to curse.

I glance at the clock. 9:15. Shit, time crawls sometimes. I hate crib today. But at least I don't have to talk recovery or AA.

I put down the Jack of spades. Dana will be here in less than two hours.

Brad snaps down a five and barks "Fifteen for two" and stabs his red peg two holes forward.

I lay down my five of hearts and mutter "Twenty for two" and slide my blue peg beside Brad's on the board. 9:21.

I can't wait for Dana to show up. And neither can Harold. When Dana first started calling on the house phone, it was Harold that picked up. He fell in love with the sound of her voice.

"She sounds hot, man," he said. "When you weren't here she talked to me for twenty minutes." Did he exaggerate, or did Dana play him? Both are distinct possibilities.

Now he's hanging around, hoping to catch a glimpse of the object of his desire.

Harold entered Fresh Start about a week before I did. Loud, obnoxious and rude, he is one of those guys everybody loves to hate. Men avoid him. He always takes more than others at meal times — not exactly an endearing quality when everyone fights for his share. It's hard to be anyone in this house, but it must be especially hard to be Harold.

"Mike, I've got your woman on the phone." Harold bounces into the room. He is almost as excited as I am. I jump up, bound through the day room and kitchen to the coffee area, and pounce on the house phone.

"Hello, Mr. Pond," Dana purrs. "I'm just down 16th Street waiting for you. Hurry up."

I dash out of Fresh Start into the cold, off the property and down the back lane and spy the little Miata, out of impound at last. I sprint to the car and fling open the passenger door. For just one moment, my life is perfect. Dana wears jeans and a red puff parka, her lips painted the exact same shade of red.

"Hello, Mr. Pond." Dana leans over and plants a vodka-laced kiss. "I can't stay long. I just needed to see you. I'm heading home for Christmas. I miss my kids so badly. I have to see them."

A can of Rockstar Mocha energy drink perches in the cup holder.

My hopes sink. "I thought you came to get me out of this place. You're drunk."

"Mr. Pond," Dana chuckles. "I'm always drunk. I've lost my home, my kids, my job. Who wouldn't drink?"

I love drunks. Someone else is always responsible for our drinking.

I try to negotiate with Dana. "I'll get my stuff. We'll go together. I have to get out of this place."

Dana tucks a loose strand of red hair behind her ear as her head pivots my way. Her other hand grips the gear shift. Her eyes show that she's already made her decision.

"No." Her voice is cold. "I will come and get you when I get back on New Year's Day. I have to go. Get out of the car now. I have to see my kids."

I move toward her. If I get close, she will listen. If she feels my touch, she will understand. She will care. Ashamed, I hear my voice plead.

"Dana, you're drunk. It's a five-hour drive over terrible roads. You're putting yourself in danger. Your kids don't want to see you like this anyway. It's not a good idea."

"Fuck you!" Dana shoves me back. "Get out! I'm out of here." Splatters of spit strafe my cheeks. She grabs her drink, takes a long gulp and then another one.

My body slumps as I slide out of the car. I'm barely out the door when the Miata spins out and fishtails down the icy back alley to disappear around the snow-banked corner.

Disappointment and despair drag me back to Fresh Start. I fall on my bed. I have to get out of here. I have to get work. I have to get a place to live. I have to get out of debt.

"Hey, Mike. How'd it go with your old lady? Did you get lucky? Hahaha." Dangerous Doug plops down onto his bed.

"No, I didn't," I say to the ceiling. "She's an out-of-control drunk like me."

Christmas Day 2008 dawns quietly. Only a handful of us are still at Fresh Start. Most are home with loved ones. As the few remaining men sit around the dining table, kind strangers dole out a few small gifts in a little Christmas bag made up by a local church. A pair of socks. A toothbrush. Toothpaste. A candy cane. A comb. A little bottle of mouthwash — the kind with no alcohol. A couple of single-wrapped Turtles. Both are gone in an instant. I love Turtles.

On this day, the pain of separation from my family is unbearable. They are gathered not far from here, at my in-laws' in Maple Ridge.

No one calls to wish me Merry Christmas. I phone Rhonda. No answer.

The phone is in a tiny alcove in one of the dorm wings, just off the kitchen. As I sit and ponder whom to call next,

I hear the forced merrymaking in the kitchen, where AA volunteers are cooking our turkey. I make myself smaller than I already am, huddle close to the phone, hoping no one will see me if I break down.

I phone my mother. Her voice catches when she recognizes mine. She sounds careworn. With one son in a down-and-out recovery home, and my brother, Roger, drunk on the streets of Saskatoon, it's almost cruel to wish her a happy Christmas.

"I'm just glad you're safe, Michael," she says. "Everything will work out. I believe you had to get out of Penticton to get sober. There are lots of resources in Vancouver. Just get all the help you can."

"I will, Mum. Love you." We cry, swallowing our sobs to stay quiet.

Over the next few days I try to reach Dana. I don't even know if she made it to the Okanagan. No response.

New Year 2009 arrives with yet another snowstorm and still no word from Dana. I call her number every day on Tom's cellphone and get only her voicemail. Is she dead or just dead drunk?

After two weeks, my brain feels clear enough for a conversation with my Penticton lawyer, Matt Jones. As if to stress the futility of my case, he recites my charges again.

"Mike, you have numerous twenty-four-hour suspensions. Two DUIs. Driving with undo care and attention causing an accident and driving while suspended." I hear the mounting frustration in his voice. "Mike, you must return to Penticton to attend court. The defence case I would need to muster up will cost you minimum ten thousand dollars. Even then it depends on the judge. Best that you plead guilty."

"If I go to prison now, how can I start a new job? I need to get work."

"Listen, Mike. The court doesn't care about any of that.

If the judge says prison, it's prison. If you don't come to Penticton, they'll send a warrant out for your arrest. I can't keep delaying this."

"Can you postpone it for another month until I see what I can do for work? I may be able to settle for something from my wife to pay you a retainer."

"Okay," Matt sighs. "I'll tell the judge you need another month of rehab. Keep me updated."

Like Rhonda should give me any money. In fact, Eli insists I turn over to Rhonda whatever remains of our joint assets.

"Listen, guy," Eli calls everyone "guy." "It's the least you can do. The damage you've done to your family — you owe them everything. Sign it all over to your ex-wife. The Big Book says you must make amends. So do it."

In the Big Book, Step 9 suggests we make "direct amends to such people wherever possible, except when to do so would injure them or others." The premise being, after we have admitted our wrongs and the people we have harmed, we go directly to those people and make our amends. Make it right.

I agonize over this decision for weeks. The therapist part of me knows I'm in no condition to make such a life-altering choice. I know I need some money to pay off the debt and start over. Yet guilt, shame and regret insist I hand everything over to Rhonda.

There is also a practical reality. Over the last few years, I've spent any money I could get on booze. If I have access to our joint assets, there's a very real chance I will drink everything away. Based upon the complaints to my professional bodies, my licences to practise have been suspended. I am told I have no choice but to claim bankruptcy. I'm recovered enough now to know I've made a colossal mess of my life.

A letter arrives from the College of Registered Psychiatric

Nurses. I gaze at the envelope, then open it, convinced it's more bad news. I read the main paragraph once. Then again, to make sure I've read it right.

The College agrees to maintain my active licence to practise, with conditions: to see a medical addictions specialist and undergo random urine testing over the next two years. I can be a psychiatric nurse again, work I haven't done in twenty years.

Just when I think I'm truly lost and will only be able to work at Tim Hortons, as Rhonda once suggested in a moment of bitterness, this lifeline arrives. I will get a job as a nurse. I'll submit to medical monitoring, if that's what it takes.

Throughout January, I trudge through deep snow to the public library every day. I spend hours applying for every nursing job in the Lower Mainland. Then I join a group of guys shovelling the neighbours' snow, to give back to the community, as AA suggests. Often we'd get invited in for coffee or hot chocolate — into real homes, where real families lived.

As January draws to a close, I'm desperate. But luckily for me, when it comes to filling nursing positions, British Columbia is more desperate. Within several days I receive several requests for interviews. February is one interview after another, punctuated by AA meetings. I'm offered positions, but many require a valid driver's licence. That counts me out.

Finally, I interview for a front-line nursing position on an adolescent psychiatric unit (APU) at a large local hospital. The interview panel is impressed with my resumé.

They don't know I am a hopeless drunk living in a rundown recovery house. They hire me on the spot. "Can you start in two weeks?" they ask.

"I can start Monday," I blurt with relief.

I return to Fresh Start triumphant. I have a job. I have a way out of this godforsaken place. Spring is just around the corner, and so is my new life.

## 11

# HAROLD

Dangerous Doug, with a hint of envy, says, "Hey, Mike. Your drunken girlfriend has been calling here all day. Eli and Josh are pissed off. You better go talk to them."

Eli does not look up. Josh rifles through the filing cabinet beside him. He shoots me a quick glance, turns away and shakes his head.

"Doug says you want to talk to me," I say to them.

"Listen, guy," Eli says. "A job won't sober you up. And a drunken alcoholic whore will kill you."

"You gotta surrender," Josh adds. "Sobriety comes before everything. I don't know how many guys I've seen relapse after they get a job and a woman."

"Hey, guy, you may have to leave here. You're doing your own program anyway." Eli concludes with a nod of his head.

"I have to work," I stammer. "My financial situation is a disaster. Dana is my girlfriend." Although I'm not sure anymore. We haven't really talked since she did her disappearing act at Christmas.

"Your priorities are all fucked up," says Josh. "She's a cumbucket. Your head has a contract out on your ass."

"If you don't follow the program, you're outta here, guy." Eli waves me away.

I storm to my room, incensed. I hate the way Josh talks

about women. I am preparing to go back and confront him when Tom walks in, rolls his eyes, shakes his head and hands me his cellphone.

"Hello, Mr. Pond," Dana's voice floods my ear.

"Dana. Where are you? I haven't heard from you in weeks." I'm relieved she's okay, but I'm still angry that she dumped me on Christmas Eve.

Here comes Harold down the hall. I turn away. I don't want him to bug me while I'm on the phone with Dana. Before my back is completely turned, his eyes meet mine. I catch an odd mix of despair and resolution. It's disquieting, that look. He doesn't pester me to speak to Dana as he usually does. He just keeps going.

I focus on Dana and where the hell she went.

"I'm in a bad way, Mr. Pond," she says. "Christmas didn't go well."

"Where are you? I've talked to your mother and she wouldn't tell me."

Long pause.

"I'm at Blaine's," she blurts. Blaine is a cocaine-addicted alcoholic we met in detox at Creekside. I remember his gaze and how he drank her in. I remember how much she revelled in it. "His girlfriend scratched the shit out of my car. She keyed it to bits. Fucking bitch."

"What! Dana, he's a crackhead. What the hell are you doing?"

"I couldn't wait for you, Mr. Pond. I'm lonely. He makes me feel good."

The cellphone falls out of my hand. I'm so pissed at her I want to scream. I want to hurl the phone against the wall and never speak to her again. I hang up.


Fresh Start is quiet. Most of the guys have gone to the nooner AA meeting in town. Dangerous Doug prods and pokes at the wood in the fireplace. It's so cold here that guys keep piling in log upon log upon log. I sit mute at the dining-room table, head in hands. How could she do this to me? What happened to my Dana? Is it because she's a drunk? Of course it is. I know I've done things drunk that sober Mike Pond wouldn't dream of. I feel warmth radiate out from the fire. I look up to watch the flames flicker. Sparks scoot up the chimney. Maybe life close to this hearth is not so bad after all. Maybe this is all I can handle right now. I'm warm and dry and sober and just a few days away from getting back to work.

The back door slams. Panicked feet pound, frantic and fast, across the floor. Someone yells. Crying. Monk leans his girth around the little office door, irritated at the interruption. Lenny runs by me, wails and collapses in front of Monk.

"Harold killed himself. Harold killed himself."

The professional in me moves. I fly out the back door just as Guy starts to cut Harold down. Harold's body slumps, his arms dangle lifeless. He hangs by a thin yellow plastic rope secured to the top bar of the rusted swing set. The bar bows in the middle. As we guide Harold down and lay him on his back, I yell, "Call 911!"

Guy and I perform CPR. Hands clasped, I push down aggressively on Harold's chest. Guy blows into Harold's mouth in tandem with my chest compressions. Guy's face is ashen. Sweat pours from his head. I recognize that Guy is in shock, ready to pass out. His head shakes no.

"I can't," he mumbles. He slumps back defeated, his hands braced behind his back.

"Let me take over." Monk shoves him aside. His big cheeks trumpet air into Harold's pale mouth. Harold suddenly regurgitates a large amount of stomach contents. Monk gags and spews the puke onto the ground. He swipes remnants from his own mouth with his sleeve, yells "Fuck!" and takes three rapid recovery breaths. I smell feces. The body has defecated. Monk speaks haltingly. "I just did this a couple of months ago with Leon. Hanged himself in the shower."

We both look down at what I'm now sure is a lifeless body.

"Sometimes I hate this fucking place." Monk resumes breathing for Harold. Doesn't give up. Continues, in what I know is futile effort, until the paramedics arrive. By then most of the guys from the house have gathered quietly, watching from a safe distance. Like suicide is contagious. Maybe it is, in a place like this. A neighbour peers over his fence. Many of us have seen this before, most on the streets, me in my work. This kind of death is part of life for those who fight addiction and mental illness.

In November it was Leon. Leon's girlfriend had broken up with him, and his wife and small children were no longer a part of his life. He tried to be upbeat. The guys say he was charismatic and funny. He kept the house entertained. Leon was an alcoholic and, like so many men here, also mentally ill. Most likely many of the black-circled faces "no longer with us," on Eli's photo collage, were mentally ill. Suffice to say after Leon died, there was no critical incident debriefing. No grief counselling. Men who struggle to put one foot in front of the other most days, who are still processing Leon's death, now must grieve for Harold too. One suicide is bad enough. Two — brutal. A pall descends over Fresh Start.

Later that day, we learn it is the tenth anniversary of the day Harold's older sister killed herself. Harold was just thirteen at the time. She also had an alcohol and drug problem.

The house feels subdued. The level of sarcasm and abusive name-calling diminishes considerably. I suppose we should be thankful for that.


In the heavy quiet of an early March morning, I get ready for work, my first day back on a hospital ward in twenty years. I feel the anxiety rise as I contemplate the enormity of my skill deficit. Things have likely changed a lot on a ward in two decades. As I wipe the remnants of shaving cream off my face, I hear a scratching noise above me. I look up and recoil in disgust. A Norway rat the size of a black lab blinks at me from a hole in the ceiling. It slips, clinging frantically, swinging by its front claws, and drops, hitting the edge of the toilet seat before scurrying into the hallway.

Hearing my yells, several guys step out of their rooms. The rat runs up and down the hallway, eyes darting in desperate search of an escape route. One of the men grabs a broom, takes a swat and misses. The rat does a U-turn, comes careening back toward me.

"Kill it! Kill it!" the chorus shrieks.

In a reflex-like movement, I stomp with full furious force right on the rat's head. I surprise myself with my quickness, timing and accuracy. This aging alcoholic still retains some athleticism. The rat is fatally injured and thrashing around. I stomp on its head again and again in an initial act of mercy that turns into a deranged expression of repressed rage.

So much for my high-minded Buddhist leanings and the sacredness of all living things. Silence descends as several of the men stand watching me.

Sick waves of shock and remorse course through me. Who am I? What have I become? I look down at my tightly clenched fists still trembling from the outburst of violence. I will them to uncurl.

"Man! You're quick. That was a hell of a shot."

Monk blinks at me. "I think you have some unresolved anger issues."

More guilt, more shame, more regret and, damn it, yet one more amend to make, this time to God's helpless creatures.

After Harold's death, after Dana's betrayal, after my

murderous rampage on the rat, I'm desperate to get out of this place. I will never get better here. I'm convinced of that. But at least I have my job.

I finish shaving and slip into the most professional-looking clothes I could borrow. But after months on the streets and in down-and-out recovery homes, can I pull off professional?

Adam, an alumnus of Fresh Start, works in Surrey and offers to drive me to my new job each day. I am on my orientation week so I have no real duties, which is a relief. After the last week at Fresh Start, I wouldn't trust me to administer medication.

I am assigned to shadow one of the nurses each shift. After so many years of working as a sole practitioner, I love being around people, especially people who at least outwardly appear to have their shit together. I receive a warm welcome.

"What are you doing working here? I hear you were a psychotherapist for fifteen years," Kate, one of the young nurses asks me. And so the obfuscation begins.

I play cool. "Oh, I shut down my practice in the Okanagan," I say. "I relocated to Vancouver. A tough divorce."

"Well, with your credentials, I guess we won't expect to see you here very long," Kate says. "I hear you used to be a head nurse on a unit like this years ago."

I smile self-consciously. I'm a long way from being in charge of anyone.

I try to concentrate on the job at hand, but my thoughts turn obsessively to Dana. She calls every day on the house phone and even today on the unit — she now knows where I work. She is back home after three weeks of drunken insanity with Blaine. I refuse her calls. Worried about her safety and her sobriety, I called her daily for three weeks. She never picked up. She knew how bad my anxiety had become, but she was too lost in her own addiction to care. I picture her with Blaine and I'm crushed by the weight of her indifference. She was my lifeline, my only friend, my lover, my last hope for a normal life.

Finally, after her second call to the unit today, I relent.

"Hello, Dana." My hand shakes.

A rush of apology tumbles from her.

"I am so sorry, Mr. Pond. I just couldn't stay in that house any longer. My sister drove me insane," Dana babbles. "I was so drunk I didn't know what I was doing. It's a total blackout. I have found us a beautiful place. We will beat this thing together."

I'm still really hurt. But she's detoxing. Trying hard to hide the tremulous, shaky sound in her voice. Working hard to sound sober.

"I don't think I can ever forget what you've done, Dana," I say.

She fast-forwards through her new plan for us.

"We can move into the place at the beginning of the month. It's fully furnished. We don't need to get a thing for it. I have found you a little rooming house close to the hospital. You can stay there for the five days until we get in."

Living with Dana is not a good idea. When it comes to falling off the wagon, I've met my match. Neither of us can remain sober long alone, and together it's even worse. But I do think I'll go insane if I have to spend one more day at Fresh Start.

"Okay, Dana. Let's do it."

"Thank you, Mr. Pond. I'll pick you up in the morning." I can hear the smile in her voice.

# 12

# LEAVING TODAY

My last night at Fresh Start, I'm restless and sleep seems impossible.

My roommate is home on a pass. I hear my door creak open.

I'm alert now, senses hyper-aware.

Two men tiptoe into my room.

Brett walks into my room. Just inside the door, Kevin snickers behind him. Brett is a twenty-nine-year-old gangster from Surrey. His head is shaved, his body covered with tattoos. He came to the house several weeks before me. He is court-ordered for residential treatment. He makes it clear to everyone he did not need to be in this "shithole." Brett is a bully who seeks out the weak and the vulnerable. Brett's buddy, Kevin, is a nineteen-year old hyperactive boy with gel-spiked hair. He is frequently caught jerking off to porn on his smartphone. The other men torment Kevin for his sexual obsession and compulsive masturbation. Kevin doesn't care. He likes the attention. Common knowledge in the house is that Kevin is Brett's "little bitch."

"Hey, Professor. How's it going?" Brett stands over my bed.

"What are you guys doing in here?" My heart slams in my chest.

"Just came down this end of the hall for a visit," Brett whispers.

"I got a nice surprise for you, old man." Kevin has his hand stuffed down his black Nike track pants.

"Both of you — get outta here. I'm not interested in any of your sick shit." My gut flutters. My breath pumps quick and shallow through my flared nostrils. My jaw clamps down. Both hands curl into tight fists. I sit up, ready to bolt.

Brett pulls a camo-handled Buck tactical knife out his black hoodie pocket and flips the shiny blade open. I've seen him show it off.

"You'll do what we tell you, mister psycho professional." The blade glints in the low light. "I've had smart-ass fuckers like you try to shrink my head before. All they did was send me back to the joint. Called me a psychopath."

Kevin sneaks closer to the bed.

"Suck on this, Doctor Mike." He pulls his erect penis out of his track pants.

I leap out of my bed. My brain throbs, ready to explode. The veins in my neck pulsate.

I swallow dryness in the back of my throat and snarl, "Both of you — get the hell out of here."

Brett thrusts the knife up a few inches from my neck.

"Just do what we want."

"Get out of here now," I growl. "Get the hell out of my room."

In an instant, all fear evaporates, replaced by rage. *Remember what happened to the rat?* My body stands taut, ready. My glare focuses tight on Brett's grey, soulless eyes. I visualize my fist smashing his nose with full driving force.

Kevin inches even closer.

You know, this might be worth it. Not a bad way to go out. Some honour to it.

Closer now, Kevin's excitement is clearly visible.

I clench my teeth in anger and disgust that my life has shrunk to this. I cannot even call it a life anymore.

Brett and I continue to lock eyes.

"Make him do it," Kevin begs.

Long pause. I don't blink.

In slow motion, Brett's knife hand returns to his pocket. He drops his eyes.

"Let's go," he grunts. "Not tonight. This isn't over, old man."

Brett pushes a sulking Kevin out the door, his penis still exposed. They will have to take care of each other tonight.

My fists uncurl. The splenius muscles running down the back of my neck and between my shoulder blades let go. My jaw slackens. Waves of nausea break over me.

I'm wide awake now. The adrenalin rush courses through me. Several days ago, a local doctor prescribed zopiclone for sleep. I never took it, trying my damnedest to adhere to the program. Eli decrees that drugs are "only an escape, a supplement to the alcoholic addiction, a precursor to relapse." I'm not sure whether a sleeping pill qualifies as mood-altering, and thus prohibited here, but I didn't want to risk it. I hid the zopiclone in a roll of socks at the back of my top drawer.

I might get sober here in Fresh Start. But I also might get killed, having managed to get on the bad side of some very bad people. I am out of here first thing in the morning.

I pop a little blue pill and slip quickly into deep, dreamless sleep.


My eyes open. My mouth feels dry with a tinny aftertaste, a well-known side effect of zopiclone. Still in a stupor, I retrieve my hidden contraband from under my stained pillow. The fluorescent blue digits on my cellphone flash 7:18. The phone was given to me by Louie, a crackhead who'd bought a hot BlackBerry Curve with some new-found cash. He just arrived at Fresh Start last week.

I pull on my clean donated American Eagle jeans and grey Gap zip-up hoodie. Shove my feet into a pair of hand-me-down size eight Adidas and head for the kitchen, on my way out to safety and freedom and God knows what else.

Tom "Guns" bumps into me.

"I'm leaving today, Tom." I grin.

"What the hell? You just got that job at the hospital. Two months sober, man. Things are starting to come back. It's too soon to leave. You'll fuck everything up."

"My girlfriend got a place in Burnaby right by the Skytrain. We can take possession first of the month. But I'm leaving today. I got a small room in Surrey a few blocks from the hospital. I'll crash there for a few days. Twenty bucks a night."

"Holy shit, man. I don't think it's a good idea." Tom shakes his head.

"I'm not staying another night in this place, Tom. I phoned Dana. She'll be here in an hour to get me."

I packed everything into my duffel bag. I don't have much. A guy doesn't need much, I've discovered. I carry my stuff out to the foyer, where I sit and wait, duffle bag by my side, precious briefcase on my lap.

The briefcase was a present from Rhonda when I first opened my private practice after graduate school in 1995. I'd buried it deep in my duffel bag to protect it. Now it's a repository of all the evidence of my downfall: collection agency notices, letters from the bankruptcy trustee, correspondence from my professional bodies, doctors' reports, police reports, papers from the Canada Revenue Agency and the Office of the Superintendent of Motor Vehicles, lab reports and anything else that reminds me that my life has turned to shit.

I wait in the foyer by the office, close to the back door,

which faces the abandoned corner store across the street. Josh, the house manager, sits in the office doing paperwork. We can just see each other, out of the corners of our eyes. We don't speak. Maybe he's written me off. After an hour and a half, Dana's Miata pulls into the corner-store parking lot. I jump up.

As I bolt, Josh yells after me.

"You're a dead man, Mike! You're not going to make it, you know that. Money and pussy kills every drunk."

That's funny — Josh is screwing another client's mother.

"I'm leaving, Josh," I yell over my shoulder as I open the door. "I have a job and a place to live."

"You haven't surrendered yet, Mike. You'll be drunk again within a month, guaranteed. I've seen it a thousand times."

"Not me. I'm done. I will never drink again." I strut out the door, my chest puffed, my head held high. Several of the guys hang out in the courtyard and watch. Dressed in jeans and a baby blue V-neck cashmere sweater, one hand on her hip, the other resting on the hood of the car, Dana paints the kind of picture every guy here fantasizes about. Glossy red curls pinned up, lips rose red and Gucci sunglasses. I can smell citrus shampoo as I nuzzle into her neck.

"Well, Mr. Pond. How does it feel?" Dana smirks. "You're out. Fucking scumbags. Stand there in front. I want to get a picture of you. Just to remember it, and know you'll never be in this shithole ever again."

I stand in front of the main gate of the old wooden fence, one hand on my hip and the other shouldering my duffle bag. I smile wide for the camera and the watching crowd. I know leaving with Dana is a bad decision. But I'm more worried about being alone. The people I care about the most now want nothing to do with me. I fear loneliness more than I fear alcoholism.

"Come on, take it quick," I say, antsy to get going. "Let's get out of here."

We merge onto Highway 99 north to freedom. Bob Marley teases "Is this love?" on the sound system.

"Well. How does it feel, Mr. Pond? You'll crash at the little rooming house for five days and then we move into our new place on the first. It's beautiful. You're going to love it.

I gaze over at her. Dana has rescued me once again. When I checked into the Phoenix Centre, I had no money. Short of cash herself, she bought me a winter coat and new boots. She knew I'd spend a lot of time on the streets. The coat and boots are long gone, disappeared in the blur of benders.

Dana pulls into the driveway of a modest house somewhere in North Surrey. An Asian woman meets us at the door.

"I will show you your room. It's downstairs. Twenty dollars a night. Five nights: one hundred dollars in advance. No refunds. You work at Surrey Memorial Hospital, right?"

"Yes," I say.

The room downstairs is small, but tidy and clean. I obsess over the bed, perfectly dressed in a crisp new blue duvet. After I've covered myself with filthy, smelly blankets for weeks, the cleanliness makes me cry with relief. I share a kitchen and bathroom with two other men in adjacent rooms.

It is peaceful and quiet here — makes me a bit twitchy.

"This is perfect," Dana nods. "Okay, Mr. Pond, let's go get some groceries."

The local Safeway is just around the corner. We meander through the aisles picking up staples. Bread, butter, eggs, milk, cheese. It's been over two months since I've had an egg or a piece of cheese. As Dana heads to the deli section for cold cuts, I unconsciously grab a two-litre carton of fresh orange juice.

"Why orange juice, Mike?" Dana asks with a tilt of her head.

"Oh. I'm craving a glass of real juice." The carton chills my hands. "All I've had is those no-name-brand bags of crystals you mix with water. Diluted to death. Zero nutritional value."

When we leave, I notice the liquor store across the parking lot. The green and yellow neon sign glows. Open. Open. Open.

"I have to go to work," Dana says. "I'll drop you off and you can make a nice ham and cheese omelette."

Dana drops me off with the groceries and backs out of the driveway of the rooming house. As I wave goodbye, my throat constricts. I'm suffused with gratitude that she is still in my life. She rescued me from Fresh Start. She bought groceries. She's lent me money until payday. All the while I know she's struggling herself. The disappearances, the long periods of silence when I don't hear from her for weeks — I know she's drinking. Now that I'm sober, maybe I can help Dana stay sober, too.

Everything goes into the sparkling clean fridge. I pour myself a huge tumbler of juice. It's ice cold, tart and sweet. I flop on the bed and turn on the nineteen-inch flat-screen TV. Eli doesn't allow TV at Fresh Start. It distracts from recovery.

"Attraction-Distraction-Subtraction" — another one of his mottos.

The Bruins are playing the Leafs. Well, we know how this will end.

God, this juice tastes good, but freedom tastes better. No one tells me when to eat, when to sleep or what to think. No one holds a knife to my neck in the middle of the night.

Now for that omelette. Shit — I forgot ketchup. Can't have an omelette without ketchup.

I hike back the three and a half blocks to the Safeway.

There it is: a plastic squeeze bottle of Heinz. It sits upside down so you don't have to fight the ketchup out. What a brilliant idea. Why did it take them seventy-five years to figure that out? Oh. Might as well pick up another carton of orange juice. After all, I'm going to be here five days.

As I step out into the parking lot, the neon beckons again. Open. Open. Open.

My eyes open but refuse to focus. In the corner the TV flickers streaks of blue and blurs of bright orange. It sounds like TSN highlights. The audio is on steroids, blasting the results of the Canucks game. I smell burnt eggs. I grasp the edge of the bed, pull my splitting head over and behold a white plate and the charred remains of a ham and cheese omelette. Smears of ketchup and bits of half-eaten toast circle the plate. Two empty twenty-sixers of Smirnoff lie on the floor. Dead soldiers. A couple of ounces left in one. I arch my head back and hold the bottle up forever until the very last drop falls and melts on the tip of my tongue. My head aches. My brain is log-jammed in the deepest fog. I reach up gingerly, touch the right side of my cheek and jaw. There is blood on my hand. I want to go look in the mirror but —

Shit! Did I leave the stove on?

I stagger to the communal kitchen in my brand-new rooming house. Thank God, the stove is off. A wreck of dirty dishes clutters the counter and sink.

As I pass the Ikea dresser at the foot of the bed, I glance in the mirror and catch sight of a head that looks like a red and purple volleyball. Holy shit, it's mine.

Black-caked blood paints the entire side of my face and down my neck. An arrangement of deep raw scrapes and cuts highlight the wound.

I need to go to the hospital. My cellphone flashes. I need to call in to work. Have I missed any work? How long have

I been drinking? My brain rapid-fires in panic mode. I count two bottles on the floor, one under the bed. That computes to two, maybe three days.

I think I had two days off. I think I'm supposed be at work right now.

# 13

# COMING BACK

My stomach plummets.

I remember now. I was at work. I went to work drunk and was told to go home. The familiar sinking realization. Fucked up again, did you, Pond? What am I going to do?

I check the messages on my phone.

Dana. "Mike, where are you? Answer your damn phone. I *knew* you were going to drink. How could you do this to us? We have a place. We have a new start. Damn you!"

Work. "Hello, Mike. This is Odette. We have you scheduled for work today. Can you please give us a call?"

Dana. "You son of a bitch. Answer your f'ing phone. Are you dead? I hope to God you are dead, you prick!"

Work. "Hello, Mike. This is Odette from APU again. We have you scheduled for an evening shift. We haven't heard from you in a couple of days. Please call the unit as soon as possible."

Dana. "I'm drunk again thanks to you. I want to die."

Work. "Mike. Please call HR."

One day out of the recovery house and I'm drunk. Barely a week in to my new job, I'm convinced I'm fired. Dana is drunk and angry. Our new place is probably history.

I need to puke. As I stand over the kitchen sink, the landlady walks in. One hand on her hip, the other finger wags at me.

"You leave now. You drunk three days. Face very bad. You go to hospital. Then you get out."

"Okay. I'm sorry."

"You go now."

Once again I cram my duffle bag with my precious brief-case and my meagre belongings. Still half drunk, I walk the eight blocks to the hospital ER in the March drizzle. Each time a vehicle approaches, I fight the compulsion to jump in front of it. A black eighteen-wheeler accelerates toward me. It would be so easy. It would be all over.

*Clinical Notes — Mental Status Exam:*

*Patient is unshaven and has a 6 cm laceration, deep scrapes and gouges to entire left side of face and eye region. Severe swelling. Patient is agitated and restless. Speech rapid and pressured. Depressed and anxious mood. Obsessive content of thought with suicidal intent. Hopeless and despairing. Impulsive. Neurotic. Disoriented to time. Intoxicated and approaching withdrawal. Poor concentration and easily distracted. Impaired insight and judgment. Diagnosis: Alcohol Dependence. Major Depressive Episode. Generalized Anxiety Disorder. Global Assessment of Functioning: 45/100. Plan: Hospitalization for medical treatment and detoxification.*

The hospital ER overflows. Old men groan and babies cry. Beds line the walls, packed with the sick and injured. After registering, I sit and watch the large digital clock in the waiting room, from 7:03 to 9:19. It's dark and raining outside.

Creekside and the Phoenix Centre are two blocks around the corner. The adolescent psychiatric unit where I work (worked?) is just down the corridor in the south wing. Minutes become hours. Hospital ERs work on triage systems. Drunks fall lower and lower on the list of priorities. At eleven p.m., I walk out.

I head for the bus stop. I have no choice. I have to go back to Fresh Start and Eli's and Josh's self-righteous "we told you so." They are right. They told me so.

The bus arrives with the hiss of air brakes. I present the driver with eighty-seven cents. With a twitch of the corner of his mouth, he allows me on. Although I know I'm a sight, in North Surrey an old guy with a smashed face reeking of liquor is not novel.

All buses smell of diesel and vinyl. I add not-so-stale booze to the mix. I lean my head on the window and watch the wet stream of coloured lights drift by. Images of Eli's face taunt me.

"Hey, guy, I told you you'd relapse. You won't surrender. Your ego will kill you."

Why hasn't his ego killed *him*? Shame and self-loathing fill me.

My downward descent into extreme alcoholism began in the spring of 2005. That's four years ago now. I've fought countless times to stay sober. And I always lose.

Begrudgingly, I recognize that I have to thank Eli. Without him, without his innate understanding of how guys like me tick, I'd have nowhere to go. If Eli takes me back, it's because he knows exactly what it's like to be me. He's been there.

I'm dying for a drink.

The bus drops me at the stop by the corner store by Fresh Start where Dana took my picture.

"Just to remember it, and know you'll never be in this shithole ever again."

I will actually be lucky to be in this shithole again. Eli may not take me back. I limp, defeated, into the house. It's just past midnight. My head and face throb with pain. Dan, the night watchman, sits sentry alone in the kitchen foyer listening to Pink Floyd's *Dark Side of the Moon* on his Sony portable. The crooked chrome telescope aerial refuses to stay upright. *Dark Side of the Moon* dissolves in a wave of static. He double-takes as I sit down.

"Holy shit, Mike." His mouth hangs open. "What happened to you? Your face is a mess."

"Don't know, Dan. Woke up this morning from a three-day drunk and this is what I saw in the mirror."

"You better lie down. Let's make up the couch of willingness outside. It's wet and cold out there, but that's where Eli will want you. I hope he lets you stay. You just left a few days ago."

"Yeah, I know. I really screwed up."

Dan and I make up the couch of willingness in the smoking pit. The area is roughly roofed in, like an old porch. Heavy clear plastic hangs on three sides to keep out the wind and rain. It's not very effective tonight. The couch is cold and wet. I pull the old blankets up to my eyes. No crisp blue duvet here. The weight of the blankets hurts the raw spots on my face.

I can't believe I'm back on the couch of willingness. Barely a week ago, I strutted out of the house in defiance, saying, "I'm ready to go." The insistence of the down-and-out Greek chorus of fellow Fresh Start clients could not drown out my confidence.

Going out, coming back, picking up, relapse. There's no end of words to refer to the essential challenge of the alcoholic — establish a period of sobriety and then, just when things get going good, you sabotage yourself.

I have one solace: Brett and his creepy sidekick Kevin have moved on.

I bat the disgusting pillow onto the floor and shiver under the pile of ancient blankets. Involuntary tremors start in my sternum and rattle out through my arms and legs. Withdrawal and the damp chill partner up. Detox begins. How long will I be on the couch of willingness this time? Dan arrives with the familiar pink plastic pail and sets it on the concrete floor beside my head.

"Hang in there, Mike. You'll be okay in a few days. If they let you stay. You were only gone a few days."

# 14

# CRAZY MIKE

I lie on this new couch of willingness as withdrawal pounces. It's the worst this time. I say that every time, but this time it really is. I wretch. My teeth chatter uncontrollably. It's impossible to get warm. The fear of another seizure grips me. The rain pounds on the porch plastic. I'm immobilized in pain for six days, punctuated by visits from the men as they pop out to smoke.

"You really fucked up, Mike," says Dangerous Doug as he sinks into an ancient chair on the porch and inhales deeply.

"Your head's got a contract out on your ass, Mike," Josh says again.

"Sobriety comes before everything, Mike." Guy stubs out his butt in the thick 1950s glass ashtray.

"Turn your will and your life over to God," Monk nods.

"We've all done it, Mike." Tom "Guns" reminds me. "You're gonna be okay."

Eli calls me into his office. He stares straight ahead, avoiding eye contact. That means he's not angry. He smirks sanctimoniously.

"I told you you'd relapse, guy. You're an alcoholic. You're selfish and self-seeking. Have you surrendered yet, guy?" Eli taps his fingers on his desk. "If you don't, you'll die. Move in with Brad." Eli is right. I am selfish and self-seeking, and he could have turfed me. I suspect a decade of dealing with guys like me has worn off any softness Eli might have had.

Once again, I've made the cut. I've graduated from the couch of willingness.

Brad is a biker and a collector for unpaid drug debts. His weapon of choice is a metal baseball bat, very effective for smashing kneecaps and breaking forearms. He's within fingertip reach in the tiny room. I cannot sleep.

Not because Biker Brad snores. No, Brad's dead-sleep utterance is much more interesting than snoring. At the transition from inhale to exhale, when his inflated lungs shift to expel air, his voice box makes a sharp, loud ping, like a WWII German submarine sonar searching for depth charges in the still night of the deep, dark English Channel. My very own *Das Boot*.

Each ping echoes through the halls of the former old folks' home. It stops at random. Ah, there, it's stopped. But no, it starts again, and again I jerk alert. Night after night.

I want to kill Brad.

I want him to kill me.

I want to kill me.

I claw at the head of the stinky, stained mattress, hanging on to life and wishing for death.

The room is dark and claustrophobic. But not dark enough. My eyes refuse to stay closed. They burn and sting. My jaw aches continuously from anxious teeth-grinding. Normally, this far along in withdrawal, I'm through feeling hyper-anxious and hyper-vigilant. This time is different and frightening.

I cannot sleep. If I do, I'll suffocate.

The struggle for breath and the compulsion to scream rise in my throat. This mental war rages the entire first night and continues for fourteen successive nights. When I slip into blessed unconsciousness, utter panic takes over. I envision being in front of a firing squad, waiting for the order to fire. I jolt awake, bathed in sweat, fearfully scanning the room.

Sleep-deprivation psychosis slithers in, and I sink deeper into delusional paranoia. My raw, damaged brain jangles.

The guys in the house hate me.

They're laughing at me.

They want me to die.

They think I'm crazy.

Another Fresh Start client, Ted, suffers from drug-induced psychosis. He's here because the courts sent him to rehab as part of his sentence.

"You're an undercover cop, aren't you, Inspector Pond?" Ted corners me in the hall. "You're a narc and you're out to bust me."

We feed into each other's delusions. I believe Ted will kill me in my sleep.

But that's no problem. I don't sleep.

Am I an undercover cop?

*Clinical Notes — Mental Status Exam:*

*Patient is underweight and undernourished. Hair unkempt and unshaven. Healing wound on left side of face. Poor hygiene and halitosis. Walks with a shuffle with head down and avoids eye contact. Facial twitches. Picks at open sores on scalp. Chews on lower lip covered with herpes. Speech low and mumbled. Mood severely depressed. Fearful and very anxious. Tense and agitated. Poor sleep and appetite. Affect depressed. Auditory hallucinations. Obsessive content of thought. Suicidal ideation. Paranoid and persecutory delusions. Impulsive. Psychotic symptoms present. Disoriented to time. Poor memory and concentration. Insight and judgment impaired.*

*Global Assessment of Functioning: 30/100 — serious impairment. Requires medical and psychiatric care. Folie à Deux.*

Folie à deux, or shared psychosis, is a psychiatric syndrome in which symptoms of a delusional belief are transmitted from one individual to another. Ted's delusions have become mine. In the middle of the night, I rummage around and search for my hidden badge and gun.

I pace the hallways, wring my hands, pick my scalp raw, chew my cold-sore-infested lip and mutter to someone or something not there. Head down, I avoid all contact. Random guttural groans escape me Tourette-like. From a clinical perspective, these utterances are supposed to diminish the anxiety. It doesn't work.

In a rare flash of insight, I know I'm not just having a bad withdrawal. The years of alcoholism have taken their toll. Abused for so long, my brain's neurotransmitters no longer know how to fire properly. I'm mentally ill, suffering from a mood disorder and probably psychosis. This is all too common among addicts. Sixty percent of those suffering from addictions also have a mental illness. Now I'm one of them. Perhaps this is what happened to some of the black-circled guys on Ed's photo collage?

Death becomes a viable option. Tonight, Biker Brad with the submarine ping is away on a pass. I cannot stand being inside my head any longer. I get up and scan the room.

Our beds stand exactly thirty-eight inches apart. I know — I measured it one day with the tape measure out of Brad's toolbox. My side of the room has a small wooden dresser at the foot of the bed. The dresser holds a limited selection of donated clothes. My duffle bag and briefcase are stowed under the bed. Brad's stuff infiltrates my side of the room. Work boots, power tools, tool belt, chainsaw, motorcycle parts, a yellow gas tank from a Harley Fat Boy. On Brad's side, the one closet holds leathers, Daytons and an uncountable array of blue jeans.

I open and shut all the drawers in the ancient dresser. I can't find what I need. I open the closet door. A quick scan of Brad's clothes, and I find it.

I pull the belt from his navy blue terry bathrobe and clove-hitch one end to the wooden bar in the tiny closet. I slipknot the other around my neck. I stand on a toolbox on the closet floor and cinch the belt snug.

To be or not to be? The inner debate is brief. My addled brain no longer possesses the cognitive ability to marshal any argument, pro or con.

I drop, almost to my knees suspended, and my airway cuts off; now, at the threshold of unconsciousness, my legs bicycle. The higher functioning part of my brain wants me dead, but the reptilian amygdala fights for survival. Flight-or-fight kicks in.

I paw at the bar to untie the tightened knot, and hang by the elbow over the bar. The slackened slipknot finally eases open and air hisses in to my body. I loosen the clove hitch and fling the belt off my neck. I collapse on the floor.

For days the telltale bruise on my throat displays another sign of my insanity. My neck is stiff and sore. If I hold my head bent slightly sideways, the pain eases.

"Did you try to off yourself, Pond?" Guy taunts me in the dining room. "You crazy fuck. Don't let Eli see that. That's all we need is another shitty corpse to cut down."

Every night, my vocal tics worsen. The noise wakes Biker Brad and he yells at me in the night.

"You're crazy, Pond. Shut the fuck up. I'm trying to sleep and you're thrashing around like a fuckin' lunatic. They're gonna lock you up in the psycho ward." He holds his filthy pillow over his head to shut me out.

I lay there silent and yell back in my head. I *am* a fuckin' lunatic, you psychopathic prick.

Brad moves to the only empty bed left — the couch of willingness. He needs his sleep, he mutters as he storms out of the room.

Everyone avoids me. Even the house management avoids me. I'm a pain in their asses. And maybe they're scared. Another casualty; another tragedy; another failure; another black circle on Eli's collage. I keep my gaze down. Every time I look up, I'm stunned that I'm here. I can't bear to look at the humanity around me.

I don't eat. I can't read. I won't leave my room except to attend the mandatory AA meetings, and when I do, I sit there mute. I'm afraid to speak because everything comes out crazy.

I hear Josh waddle my way. He stands in my doorway, one hand on his hip, the other stretched over his head, resting on the door frame.

"Your work called, Pond." Josh looks at me with distaste. "It's been two weeks. You better call them. Your whore called, too. Don't you dare call her! I told you a job and a woman would take you out. Sobriety has to come before everything."

This is standard recovery-house language — women's value expressed as only sexual, in the crudest possible language. Dana is not a whore or a cumbucket — that's the worst one. She is my last connection to my previous life. But I no longer have any fight left in me to tell Josh off.

I drag my feet to the office and dial work.

"Hello, Odette. It's Mike Pond. I'm sorry I haven't been to work. I have been very sick."

"We haven't heard from you, Mike. I have talked to HR and management. You have to meet with the occupational health nurse. She'll assess you and recommend a plan."

"I haven't been fired?" I am incredulous.

"I don't know. I've never dealt with anything like this before. You are on a leave without pay at this point. You barely started your three months' probation. Mike — do you have a drinking problem?" Odette asks bluntly.

"No," I lie.

"Have you seen a doctor?" Odette sounds suspicious. "You have to get a doctor's note."

"No, I haven't. I will. Thank you, Odette."

Josh nods self-righteously as I hang up. He recites by rote from the Alcoholics Anonymous Big Book (page 58): "Rarely have we seen a person fail who has thoroughly followed our path. Those who do not recover are people who cannot or will not completely give themselves to this simple program, usually men and women who are constitutionally incapable of being honest with themselves. There are such unfortunates. They are not at fault; they seem to have been born that way. They are naturally incapable of grasping and developing a manner of living which demands rigorous honesty. Their chances are less than average."


Josh chauffeurs me to the walk-in medical centre on 152nd Street. A sign shows up in several strategic places throughout the clinic: "We do not write prescriptions for narcotics or other controlled medications." Drug abuse runs rampant in this quaint little seashore town, home to millionaires and retired police officers.

Dr. Holic steps into the examination room. He's a kind-hearted man who speaks with a strong Czech accent. I saw him once before, when I first arrived at Fresh Start. A lot of the men see him. Back then he gave me a physical exam, wrote a prescription for my thyroid medication and scratched a brief note for social assistance saying I couldn't work because I was in treatment for severe alcoholism.

"What can I do for you today, Mr. Pond? Your lab results

from a few months ago look fine." Dr. Holic flips through my chart.

"I need a medical note from you for my employer, saying I'm sick."

"What's wrong with you?" He looks up from the chart.

"I told them I have an infection."

"What kind of an infection? Take off your shirt and sit up here." He gestures to the exam bed and I hop up. Dr. Holic places his stethoscope on my chest. He shakes his head. He's seen a lot of drunks and alcoholics.

"Did you start drinking again?" he asks.

Long pause.

"If I don't get a note saying I'm really sick, I won't get my job back. I barely started my probationary period." I stare at the floor.

"Mr. Pond, you are sick. Very sick. You have a disease. It's called alcoholism. I will write you a note and it will say exactly that. You have an illness and you require treatment. You need a medical leave."

"They'll fire me."

"I will agree to monitor you medically." He scribbles a note.

"Thank you, Dr. Holic. But I think I'm done."

"Mr. Pond, you just have to get well. That's the only thing that matters right now." He tears off the note and hands it to me. It says I need a medical leave because I am an alcoholic.

I return to the house. Josh hands me an envelope. It's been opened. Bastards read my mail. The letterhead reads Fraser Health Human Resources.

I must complete a medical assessment by a qualified addictions specialist at my own personal cost. The College of Registered Psychiatric Nurses and the College of Registered Social Workers concur with my employer. I must have the assessment before the hospital will even consider my return to work. But I know these assessments are expensive — around fifteen hundred dollars, as I recall. I stare at the collage of black-circled men, convinced it's just a matter of time until I'm up there with them.

Where the heck am I going to get that kind of money?

"Looks like you're screwed, eh, Pond?" Monk says nonchalantly.

Desperate, like a candidate on a game show I call all my lifelines.

"Mum, I have a chance to keep my job if I get a medical assessment by an addictions specialist, but it will cost fifteen hundred dollars."

"Mike ..." Her voice sounds quiet and sad. "I just do not have that kind of money."

I know she does. She also has a long history of lending money to drunks.

Then my ex-wife, Rhonda.

"Mike, even if I had the money, I wouldn't give it to you."

Finally, my step-mum. The answer is the same.

My last phone call, to Odette at the hospital. Since Dr. Holic refused to lie for me, I have no choice.

"Odette, when you last called, I didn't tell you the truth." I twist the phone cord in my free hand. "Yes. I am an alcoholic."

Odette sighs. "Mike, I don't like being lied to. If HR allows you to continue your probation period, you'll have to be medically monitored."

I hang up.

Eli chimes in. "They will never take you back. You fucked up in your first week of a new job. What sane employer would hire a sick fuck like you."

As if in a trance, I trudge the long hallway to my room and plunge face first onto the bony mattress. I surrender. This is my fate — recovery houses, welfare, washing dishes at the Boathouse Restaurant. Pay off the bottle of Scotch I owe them.

I play crib. It passes the time, and it's about the only sanctioned recreation going. We're not allowed to go to the gym — it's a waste of time that should be devoted to working the steps of AA. More than that, according to Eli, pumping iron feeds our already gargantuan egos.

I miss going to the gym. When I was particularly stressed and exhausted after a day of counselling my most troubled clients, I could feel my anxiety dissipate with each rep.

I can't concentrate. I deal the cards, hoping for some fives and tens. It's easier to count fifteens. Angry Gord is my partner today. He's a long-time AA volunteer who sponsors many of the guys who come and go through Fresh Start. Gord was once a raging alcoholic convicted of spousal assault. He was ordered to see Dr. David Acres, an expert in the medical treatment of addicts, himself a twenty-year-sober prescription drug addict. Dr. Acres helped Gord finally quit drinking, but Gord remains angry. When a guy gets a nickname around here, it tends to stick for a reason. Angry Gord. Crazy Mike.

Angry Gord holds a certificate in addictions counselling. His efforts to get into the counselling business have failed miserably. He is, however, a master crib player. While I update him on the sorry state of my affairs, he kicks my ass. Then he makes an astoundingly generous offer.

"I'll give you the money, Mike." He looks up from his cards. "You're a professional. You've got to get back to work. You don't have to pay me back. Consider it my investment in our partnership. We'll be making damn good money in the future. With your credentials and my experience, it's a no-brainer."

Repeatedly, reluctantly, I turn down his offer. I can't

possibly take that kind of money from a near stranger. But I have no choice.

"Okay, Gord. I will pay you back when I can, though. Thank you."

Dr. Acres' medical monitoring costs fourteen hundred dollars. Paid in full with Angry Gord's money, I book my two-and-a-half-hour session. I'm scheduled to go in on April Fool's Day. I can't quite kick the unease I feel about taking Angry Gord's money.

Monk drives me to my first appointment. I am sick with worry. I've been taking zopiclone, the medication that Dr. Holic prescribed for sleep. The latest research reports that it is just as addictive as benzodiazepines, which are used to treat anxiety. Paranoia convinces me that the lab tests will detect the zopiclone. I'll be out. I cannot — cannot — waste this lifeline.

"I've really screwed up, Monk," I confess from the passenger seat on our way to my appointment. "I won't be able to work ever again. They'll take my licence to practise away forever."

"Settle down, Pond. It's going to be okay. Just sit there and relax. We're almost there." Monk's eyes dart my way and back, aware of the traffic and me at the same time.

"Stop the car," I say, my hand on my seatbelt buckle. "Let me out. I can't go for this assessment."

Monk breathes harder and more loudly now. He grips the steering wheel, as if willing me to stay in the van. My fear and panic become unbearable. The mad desire to run overtakes me.

"Pull over here. I want out!"

Monk pulls over in a residential area. I bolt out of the van and race up the street. Monk flies out of the driver's side, just avoiding a passing truck. The driver honks. Monk bears down on me like a linebacker and tackles me at the hips. Shit,

I forgot just how agile the big bastard is. The wind oomphs out of me and I slam face first into someone's front lawn. Monk hoists me effortlessly over his shoulder back to the van. I've lost some serious weight in the last several months.

"Get in!" he slams me into the seat. "Don't move till we get to the doctor's office. I mean it!"

The shock jolts me into temporary sanity and submission.

"Okay," I nod. "I will."

The waiting room in Dr. Acres' office is large. Several men and women sit in it, reading magazines.

"Michael Pond?"

An assistant stands by the reception desk with my file. I follow her into the examination room and wait for my fate.

Dr. Acres enters. His hair is salt-and-pepper. His warm eyes size me up, eyes wizened by experience. These are eyes of a long-recovered addict.

"Hello, Mr. Pond. I see we are doing a full assessment for Fraser Health and the College of Psychiatric Nurses. Before we start, I need you to go down to the lab and give a urine sample. Then I will ask you a battery of questions. In one week, I will have you come back and we will review my report."

Dr. Acres waits for me in the examination room while I give my sample.

"Sit down, Mr. Pond," he says when I come back. "Try to relax. I see you're very anxious. How long have you had a drinking problem?"

"I think I was born an alcoholic. My father is a recovered alcoholic. My grandfather died due to alcoholism. My brother is an alcoholic."

"So you know you have a genetic predisposition?"

"The last five years have been very bad. I've lost everything: my career, my home, my family ..."

Dr. Acres nods. "All this can come back," he says. "Let's continue."

I offer a synopsis of my life with alcohol: the family history, culminating in the final train wreck with Dana.

He listens with a look that says "I've heard this before. A lot."

"Mr. Pond, you have a tragic story," he says. "You have a progressive illness, and it will only get worse if you don't maintain an effective treatment program for the rest of your life. I know I'm not telling you anything you don't already know, but I can't be more adamant. You will definitely die if you don't stop drinking. Quite frankly, I'm utterly amazed you've made it this far. However, with an absolute commitment to recovery, you can get your life back. Maybe not like it was or how you want it, but it will come back."

I am not convinced. I am also not being completely truthful. I know I should reveal my suicidal thoughts, but then Dr. Acres will be forced to say I'm too ill to go back to work. And going back to work is my salvation.

15

# ROCK BOTTOM

"Mike, your ex-wife phoned again," says Monk.

"Mike, you have a letter here from the Canada Revenue Agency," says Eli.

"Mike, some collection agency keeps calling here looking for you," says Joe.

"Mike, there's a bunch of mail from Visa and MasterCard on your bed," says Brad.

"Mike, your lawyer called," says Josh.

The banks have found me, along with all my other creditors. I am in serious trouble. That's funny — as if I wasn't in serious trouble already.

The top drawer of my tiny dresser overflows with their demands. They all want money I don't have.

After my unexplained no-show a week on the job as a psychiatric nurse, I'm convinced I don't have a job anymore, either. I don't believe the assessment will save me. It will only confirm what I already know: I am unredeemable. I've collected enough alcohol-related criminal charges to know that I face doing serious time. I feel an all-pervasive sense of doom.

Last week, Dr. Acres prescribed me trazodone. It's a non-addictive antidepressant used for sleep. It's not working. Since I left his office nine days ago, I haven't slept. Worry worms deep into my thoughts. All the jumbled, jangled, tortured tendrils weave together nonsensically and coalesce into a monstrous ball of anxiety.

I'm trapped. I see no way out. I'm convinced Dr. Acres' report will be bleak. It will conclude that I'm a lying drunk with no hope of rehabilitation, unfit to work as a health care professional ever again. It will sentence me to a lifetime of recovery houses and group homes. Not even Tim Hortons will hire me. I will be forced to file for bankruptcy. Rhonda will keep our house. My sons will never talk to me again.

I refuse to leave my room. Biker Brad has permanently relocated to the couch of willingness. I don't blame him. I'd walk a wide berth around me.

Alone at night, the voices echo raspy and metallic, as if they come from a transmitter.

*You're a fuck-up. Kill yourself. Kill yourself. Kill yourself.*

They whisper from the heating vent.

*You useless piece of shit! Look what you've done. You're better off dead.*

My head ricochets. They jump to the closet.

*You're a liar, a cheat and a thief. You deserve to die. Do everybody a favour and hang yourself. You can't even do that right, loser.*

Oh yes I can. I squirm out of bed and yank on my hand-me-downs. They haven't been laundered in over a month.

I sneak out the back patio door into the cold, wet spring night. The dining-room clock reads 1:53. Dan, bobbing his head to his Sony, doesn't notice me.

"The years rolled slowly past, and I found myself alone."

Bob Seger's "Against the Wind." Appropriate tonight.

I hit Marine Drive and veer west past the fish-and-chip joints, swimwear shops and ice cream parlours. As I walk, an easy peace envelops me.

Half-hearted moonlight bathes the silent shops. A police

cruiser coasts up from behind. The officer glances my way and drives on. I'm just a little old man on a late-night walk.

Just before the famous White Rock Pier, I hike down to the beach. At high tide, White Rock Beach isn't much of a beach at all. A vast, still sea of boulders beckons me, craggy shapes silhouetted in the blue moonlight. The waves whisper behind them.

I spot a rock about the size of a shot put. I hoist it up into my arms. It weighs about fifteen pounds. With the rock braced on my groin, I trudge stiff-armed up the bank and sway down the long wooden pier. The dim bulbs strung overhead glow with ghostly light, reminiscent of a Van Gogh painting.

My wasted arms complain under the rock's dead weight. How I wish I had a bottle.

I reach the end of the pier, where the water is deepest. I heave the rock up to rest on the rail at my chest. I finger initials carved into the wooden rail over the years, imagining long-ago lovers on a warm, sunny day, sea wind lifting their hair. Their laughter and intimate murmurs mingle with the squawk of greedy seagulls circling above.

The black water laps against the creaking pier, pulling me back to this moment. Boat masts squeak and sway in harmony with the waves.

Balancing the rock with one hand, I swing myself up to sit on the handrail. My feet lock behind the lower bar. I roll the stone anchor into my lap and peer over my knees. The inky water coaxes below, rolling in soft swells. I undo my belt, slide the rock inside the front of my pants and zip up over it. I stare down into the deep water. I hate cold water. I teeter forward and my feet hook more tightly under the lower rail. My hands grip the front rail by my hips, the worn wood biting splinters into my palms.

No more mental torment. No more taunting voices.

I imagine my dead, bloated body floating on the surface.

I remember boating to the cliffs at the southeast end of Skaha Lake. Brennan's body curled in a ball as he catapulted off that sixty-foot wall of granite.

He crashed into the water, burst above the waves, screaming, "Did you see that, Dad? Pretty awesome, eh?"

I imagine myself under the waves, clawing at the water in a frantic struggle to reach the surface as the rock in my pants sinks me to the depths and eternity.

I teeter on the fence. I shut my eyes and breathe in the April mist, the ocean air, the stillness of the pier. My hands quiver on the rail.

Shit.

My boys. Taylor smiling big and toothy, his broad, square Nordic chin. Brennan excitedly telling a story of his latest camping trip at Sawmill Lake. Jonny running down the rugby pitch with his short, thick legs pumping.

I unzip my pants, hoist the rock up and watch it plummet into the water.

I'm such a chickenshit. Suicide is harder than I thought.

I plod back to Fresh Start. Another failed attempt.

I need a gun. I compile a mental list of the guys who might have guns. I suspect Anton has a Glock stashed. Maybe that street punk, Colin? Amir has one for sure. He threatened to blow Eli's fucking head off one day.

When I return to my room, the voices announce their verdict.

*Loser. Coward. Knew you couldn't do it.*

Insight can be a curse. I'm psychotic and I know it. Most of the time.

*Clinical Notes — Mental Status Exam:*

*Patient has poor hygiene, with soiled clothes and body odour.*

*Psychomotor agitation and restlessness. Low, whispered speech. Mood depressed and anxious. Affect blunted. Hypervigilant. Insomnia. Auditory hallucinations. Obsessive-compulsive traits. Paranoid and persecutory delusions. Suicidal ideation and intent. Poor concentration and distractible. Judgment poor. Insight good. Global Assessment of Functioning: 35/100 — Major impairment.*

The early morning hours tick by. Sleep visits for no more than ten minutes at a stretch. For several days, anxiety immobilizes me.

I call and postpone my visit with Dr. Acres. I'm too afraid to leave my room.

April the eighth dawns grey and rainy.

Rhonda drives down to Vancouver with her boyfriend. At my request, she contacted a lawyer and asked him to draw up the papers so I can sign my one remaining asset — our home, held jointly — over to her. Signing over the home means accepting I'll never live there again. I've always held out hope that someday I would recover and I'd be invited back.

I'm sober but a long way from recovered. I'm sick with anticipation of this next loss. Perhaps signing over everything is another mistake? Even Eli, who is big on making amends, isn't sure this is the right thing to do. "Yah, guy, it's the right fuckin' thing to do. Least you can do," is what he said yesterday. But today, he quietly approached me and said he wasn't sure he'd given me the right advice.

This time, Josh drives me to the lawyer's office. Rhonda found him through the Yellow Pages. I just needed a lawyer to witness the deed.

We wait in the parking lot.

It's been a while since I've seen Rhonda. I study myself in

the car mirror, and for the first time in a long time, I really see myself. Face still covered with cold sores. Gaping wounds in my scalp where I scratched worry holes. I look like an old man as I gum my lip.

Rhonda's green CRV pulls into the parking lot. Her new partner ducks out with the dog as Rhonda waves me into the car. She chatters in her matter-of-fact way, as if we're going to Costco to do the family shopping. Only we're signing away the last dregs of my life. I tremble with agitation, my anxiety amplified by the situation. My memory jets back twenty-five years to Thanksgiving, the day Rhonda first introduced me to her family as the man she wanted to marry.

She led me by the hand up the walkway to the main door of her parents' sprawling rancher. I noticed an embroidered plaque: "I am the way and the truth and the life. No one comes to the Father except through me. John 14:6 (NIV)." I was met first by the royal family. Plaques and pictures of Queen Elizabeth II, Prince Philip, King George VI, the Queen Mother and the newly married Prince Charles and Di jockeyed for space. Rhonda smiled.

I trailed her into a Norman Rockwell painting. Three pumpkin pies sat on the counter waiting for whipped cream. I peeked in the oven and a waft of hot, savoury air hit my face and fogged my glasses. Extra sausage-meat stuffing wrapped in tinfoil lay on the oven rack beside the big blue roasting pan. Elaine, Rhonda's older sister, was mixing two big bottles of ginger ale into a crystal punch bowl. Alcohol-free. In the family room the open wood fireplace crackled. Rhonda's father, Armond, sat on the couch playing his banjo and singing "Somewhere in Heaven."

Rhonda introduced me shyly and proudly. "This is Mike, Dad."

I was in heaven.

Armond placed the banjo at his side, pushed himself up,

limped across the room, let out a deep belly laugh, grabbed my arm and shook it like he was shaking off an old dirty carpet. That was the beginning of one of the most satisfying and grounding relationships of my life. I was besotted with Rhonda, but in Armond I found unconditional love. Here was a man rooted in his family. Rhonda's mother was unwavering in her Christian beliefs. She said, "If you want to be with our daughter, you need to turn your life over to the Lord and become a Christian." So I did. I found stability in their world of absolutes. I gave my life to the Lord Jesus Christ. I was baptized in water and in the Holy Spirit. I became a believer, even a Sunday-school teacher.

After I asked Rhonda to marry me, my friend Billy took her aside and said, "Maybe you should think this through, Rhonda. You know Mike has a drinking problem." For a long time in my marriage, I didn't have a drinking problem. Choosing Rhonda, becoming part of her family, inoculated me against being a drunk.

It appears I needed a booster shot.

Twenty years later Rhonda would say to me, "I should have listened to Billy." When I think of how much I've disappointed Armond and hurt his daughter, tears well. I wipe my eyes and push the car door open. "Let's go in and get this thing over with."

As Josh, Rhonda and I file into the office, the lawyer eyes me carefully.

"Mr. Pond. I want to make it very clear you are not getting legal counsel from me." He speaks slowly, hitting every consonant. "You have no legal counsel here. I am just witnessing your signature. Is that clear?"

What's clear is that he's questioning my mental state.

I sign the documents. We leave.

Josh drives me back.

"It was the right thing to do," he says to the windshield.

I rest my head against the cool window. The fog from my breath obliterates the outside world. I don't know what the right thing is anymore. I have no legal assets. I am officially destitute. The car rolls along the road back home to Fresh Start.

# 16

# I'M DONE

A week goes by and I have barely left my room, but today I must. Today, Dr. Acres will deliver his report. He'll share it with me first, then he'll deliver it to the authorities. I need to show up at his office, even though I know it will all end badly. Monk offers to drive me. He's taking all the guys downtown for the North Shore Round-Up, a renowned AA event held every year in Vancouver. Thousands of alcoholics gather for a weekend of dry fun — a contradiction in terms if there ever was one.

I must play normal for the doctor, particularly this doctor. He holds my shaky future in his hands.

I'm actively suicidal. Dr. Acres knows — based on a search of the database where all the province's prescriptions are logged — every medication that's been prescribed to me over the last five years. He suspects I have a history of misusing benzodiazepines. He must know I've been taking zopiclone on the sly at Fresh Start. But the stuff doesn't even work.

Dr. Acres greets me in the exam room.

"Good day," he says, and smiles. "You look rough today. Are things okay?"

"Yeah, I'm fine," I shrug. "Ready to go back to work. I need to go back to work. A lot of debts to pay right now."

"Well, your lab work came back negative." Dr. Acres taps my chest. "However, your prescription report shows a lengthy history of taking benzodiazepines and hypnotics."

My shoulders drop with relief. The zopiclone wasn't detected. It appears that not everyone is against me.

"I have taken Ativan," I explain, "and other anti-anxiety agents over the years, for sleep and withdrawal."

He stops me. "You're poly-doctoring. You've had six different doctors over the last five years alone. It appears you have a problem with prescription medication as well as alcohol. The point being, you have a long history of alcohol and drug abuse."

I'm too wound up to articulate an argument. I know in my heart I'm just an alcoholic. I used pills over the years only to combat the effects of the booze. On my downward spiral, I only went to walk-in clinics, thus the six doctors in five years.

But really, what does it matter what kind of mess I am? I'm a mess.

Dr. Acres continues. "I'm recommending that you remain in the recovery house or a similar treatment centre for a minimum of three months. You must remain abstinent. You must attend AA meetings at least three times a week. You must provide clean random urine specimens for the next two years. You must be medically monitored by an addictions specialist. At the end of three months, if you meet all these conditions, I will recommend a gradual return to work."

A shock of relief heaves out of me. But it is short-lived.

"The monitoring will cost six hundred dollars up front," Dr. Acres says, "and you'll pay one hundred dollars each time you provide a random urine sample. The average is eighteen samples a year over the two-year period."

My broken brain does the math: $4,200. That's a pile of money that I don't have, and see no way to obtain.

I stare at a picture on the wall, of a college soccer team

surrounding the doctor, autographed by the players. On the bottom it reads "Thanks, Doctor Dave."

Inanely, I read it out loud. "Thanks, Doctor Dave."

"You're welcome. You'll need to see me every two weeks. Book your next appointment with Anna. See you then. I'll send the report to your employer and the College of Psychiatric Nurses."

Monk waits outside in the van, his massive bulk hunched over a paperback, *Awakening the Buddha Within*. Several guys from the house stand on the sidewalk. They smoke, leer and make rude gestures to women walking by.

Monk sees me, snaps the book shut and hollers, "Let's get going! We have to be at the Hyatt downtown by twelve."

I don't want to go. I want to go back to the recovery house. Forty-two hundred dollars might as well be a million. After the finality of signing over my one remaining asset to Rhonda, I've lost all hope. My head rests on the passenger window. As shop windows and people blur by, the guys bombard me with ridicule.

"How's it feel getting loaded then going to work to take care of a buncha mentally ill kids, Pond?"

"Yeah, Pond. You're more fucked up than the crazies you look after."

"Hey, Crazy Mike. You're crazier than the crazies. You need bug juice. Hahaha."

They're right. I can hardly discriminate their voices from the ones in my head.

At the Hyatt, thousands of people bump and mill about. I wander amidst them, confused and disoriented.

I spy Matt Jones, my lawyer. He walks my way with a big toothy smile. No! That's not him. It can't be him. He's in the Okanagan. He's an alcoholic attending the rally? That's why he's here. No, he's here to take me to jail! I pivot and career through the crowd in the other direction. I want to jump in front of that bus.

Monk's massive paw clamps onto my shoulder. He spins me around. "Not on my watch, Pond! Get in the van. I'm taking you back, you crazy son of a bitch!"

Since he was my desperate resuscitation partner for Harold a few months ago, keeping me alive has become Monk's mission. We are like war buddies now, locked in grim camaraderie.

Monk's eyes narrow as he shoves me into the vehicle.

We race south on Highway 99. Monk's paws pinch the steering wheel of the blue '89 Chevy van. The high noon sun glares into our eyes.

Monk's moon-shaped face stares straight ahead. He pulls the visor down and with firm calmness says, "Don't even think about it, you crazy fuck, or I'll kill you myself."

That's right, I'm thinking about it. I'm thinking about nothing else. Whipping along at 112 kilometres per hour, I will simply open the door and jump out.

I unclick my seatbelt, muffling the sound with my hand, and let it retract slowly. My right hand clutches the door handle, fingers wrung tight on the chrome. If I open it quickly and fly out, it will be over fast.

"I'm done," I swallow, hard.

"Don't open that fucking door, Pond," Monk commands, keeping his eyes trained on the road. "Just relax, damn it! I'm taking you to the hospital."

My fingers squeeze the door handle until we screech to a halt at the ER entrance of Peace Arch Hospital in White Rock. Monk runs around to my side and flings open the door.

"Get out! Now!"

"I can't go in there. They'll certify me." I cannot be certified as a crazy person. Even in my advanced state of mental decompensation, I know my career as a therapist is toast if I get certified.

"You *are* certifiable, Pond. Get the hell out of the van! If you don't go on your own two feet, I will carry you in there."

Under the Mental Health Act, if I'm certified, I am deemed a danger to myself and/or others and will be legally held against my will for up to thirty days in a psychiatric facility. I don't budge.

Monk phones Josh, the house manager.

Josh's tinny voice vibrates through the phone.

"You know they don't want crazy fucks like him there," he says to Monk. "They hate drunks. You're wasting your time."

Monk is frantic. "I don't know what else to do with him. He's driving me crazy. He's going to off himself. He almost jumped out of the van." Monk glares at me.

Faced with 310 pounds of fury, all five foot six of me acquiesces. I may be crazy, I may want to kill myself, but I don't want to suffer undue pain. I go limp. As we say in mental health lingo, I decide to become compliant. For now.

Other patients smell my stale, sweaty presence before laying eyes on me. I know I look terrible. My toothbrush and I broke up a long time ago. I haven't shaved or showered in two weeks, despite constant friendly hints like "Pond, you smell like ass and look like fuckin' shit" and "Don't touch the food, Pond, you'll contaminate it." I refuse to shower. I now not only look the part, but live the part of a skid-row bum. I just don't care.

Tremors rack my body, my breath flaps shallow and rapid. My heart flip-flops in my chest. A steel band pulls ever tighter around my temples — paralyzing anxiety. Everyone stares at me.

A young couple whisper to each other and gesture in my direction.

An old man says, "Hey, buddy, would you just sit down and wait like the rest of us? There are some people in here who are really sick, you know."

Even to many health care workers, mental illness does not present with the same kind of urgency as a heart attack. But the sad reality is that addiction and mental illness can kill just as efficiently as heart disease.

After several hours, a young, blond, ponytailed nurse surveys the waiting room. Her eyes come to rest on me.

"Mr. Pond? Come with me." She leads me to an exam room and takes my vital signs. My pulse and blood pressure are through the roof.

"What brings you to Emergency today, Mr. Pond?" Her voice is calm, soothing and sympathetic.

"I'm an alcoholic. I've lost everything. I don't want to live anymore," I say.

"How much have you been drinking, and when did you have your last drink?"

By rote, I deliver every answer. I know my response to the next question will make or break this deal.

"Do you have a plan to kill yourself, Mr. Pond?"

The shred of hope I have left for my future hangs on my next words. The debilitating depression, the extreme anxiety, the paranoid delusions, the auditory hallucinations, the repeated thoughts of suicide urge me to scream yes.

And then I see myself in a Tim Hortons uniform. Oddly fitting, because Tim Horton, the professional hockey player who founded the chain, was a notorious alcoholic who killed himself by driving drunk.

As I open my mouth, Monk steps into the room.

"I want to be here for this," he says to the nurse. "This little fucker will scam you. He's smooth and he's slick."

Monk knows the medical staff, and they know he works at the recovery house. His story of redemption is legend in

135

these parts. He's also engaged to an RN in Pediatrics. He leans back in his chair. "I have seen over four hundred men come through the house over the last two years, and this guy by far is the craziest motherfucker of them all. He scares the shit out of me. He tried to jump out the van going 110. He wants to off himself."

That's it. I know at that moment that I will be pinked — sent straight up to the psych unit, stripped naked, put in pyjamas and locked in the seclusion room with nothing but a mattress, a strong blanket and a bedpan. In my past career as a psychiatric nurse, I performed hundreds of assessments myself. Now it will happen to me.

The doctor limps in, leaning on his cane.

In a strong Scottish brogue, he introduces himself.

"I'm Dr. MacIntosh. I'm the attending psychiatrist."

This is the dude, the one who signs the certificate. He holds the power. He looks to be in his mid-sixties with shaggy eyebrows. Like two miniature potted plants, thick tufts of stiff hair grow out of his ears.

He rests his cane on the arm of the chair and rattles through all the questions I've just answered.

"Do you have a plan to kill yourself, Mr. Pond?"

He and I both know I do. But I'm not crazy enough to admit it.

After fifteen frustrating minutes, Dr. MacIntosh cannot get me to say that I want to kill myself. He knows I am doing a very good job of eluding involuntary admission. He's angry and lets me know it.

"You are full of unexpressed anger, Mr. Pond," he sighs. "You are a bleeding-heart social worker from the eighties who does not trust the medical profession. I will not admit you. It is a waste of a good hospital bed."

"Thank you, doctor," I say with relief.

"I want you to tell me that you do not have a plan to kill yourself."

I lie and comply. "I do not have a plan to kill myself."

He writes me a prescription for olanzapine, a new-generation antipsychotic, and Celexa, a selective serotonin reuptake inhibitor antidepressant, and hands me one milligram of sublingual Ativan, an anti-anxiety agent. Dr. MacIntosh then snatches his cane, rises up and gingerly limps out. He pauses in the doorway.

"Good luck, Mr. Pond," he says. "You're going to need it. Most men your age whose alcoholism has progressed to the degree yours has don't make it. Or they end up spending the rest of their years in an institution."

I return triumphant to the waiting room, where Monk sits reading a magazine.

"Fuck!" He shakes his head.

By the time we return to the van, the Ativan has kicked in. My anxiety diminishes considerably. This is a highly addictive benzodiazepine that works. Trouble is, like every addictive thing, its relief is temporary and elusive.

I slump against the passenger door.

Monk fumes. I'm his problem again. But not for long — our recovery house does not take men prescribed psychotropic medications.

Monk furiously works his phone as he drives. "Hello, Randy? Do you still take guys on bug pills? Yeah, I got this guy. He's crazy and has to take psych drugs. Do you want him?" Monk drives with one hand on the steering wheel while the other cups his phone to his ear. He nods with satisfaction. A big cheesy-assed grin on his round face, he whips a U-turn and hits the gas, and we speed north on Highway 99.

"You're going to Mission Possible," he says. "I guess you're getting certified anyway. Only in a different kind of way, Crazy Mike."

# 17

# MISSION POSSIBLE

Mission Possible sits nestled in the lush farm country of South Langley, literally a stone's throw from the American border. In the distance, a low, steady hum drones from the two highways that run for miles directly parallel on opposing sides of the US–Canada border. This stretch of road is the largest illegal drug portal to Canada. Only someone with a wicked sense of irony would situate a recovery home here.

As Monk negotiates his way through the potholes of Mission Possible's long driveway, the effect of the Ativan begins to wear off. The SUV comes to rest in front of a typical nineties rancher.

Monk escorts me into the house. Where the Fresh Start feels claustrophobic, Mission Possible feels expansive. A large open foyer stretches into a spacious multi-windowed meeting room. The house office sits off the foyer.

"Hey," a six-foot-tall, lanky guy addresses me. His long neck hunches forward, cutting an Ichabod Crane–like figure. "Hear you're a shrink. Well, here you're just another fuckin' addict."

This is Randy, Mission Possible's program director.

"I run a better program here than Fresh Start." He points proudly to a large clipping from the Vancouver *Province* newspaper, framed and displayed on the wall in the main foyer for all to see. A picture shows Randy with a large grin, standing proudly on the recovery house's porch. The headline reads "Recovered Addict Devotes His Life to Helping Others."

Another guy in his late thirties, with shaggy greying hair, peers out of the office behind Randy and introduces himself.

"Hi, I'm Ken, the house manager. I'm two months clean and sober. Actually it's over a year, but I screwed up and smoked a joint a couple months ago. Ken, I soon learn, is a former heroin addict.

Two months. I have come to learn that length of sobriety is the true measure of a man in recovery.

With his usual cat-like stealth, Monk slips out of the house and backs the van out of the driveway. As he drives off, he yells out the window, "I'll get someone to bring your stuff out here later."

He can't wait to see the last of me. And I could care less about getting my belongings. Stuff is becoming less and less important to me — except for my briefcase.

"We'll transfer your welfare cheque over to Mission Possible. Now read this tenancy agreement and sign it." Randy shoves the contract my way.

Ken takes me on a tour of the home. Upstairs are three bedrooms, two for men who have graduated to a state of semi-privacy, and one for Ken. He's got the master bedroom. It's huge, with a balcony, walk-in closet and Jacuzzi tub. A massive new flat-screen TV dominates one wall.

For the foreseeable future, the dorm in the basement will be my home. I follow Ken down the narrow stairs to a large former rec room, now crammed with six sets of bunk beds. I imagine a Ping-Pong table, and a big entertainment centre on the far wall. Kids playing and laughing, now replaced by down-and-out men snoring and crying out in their tortured sleep. When the house is full, eighteen guys share two showers.

Ken assigns me a mattress on the top bunk in the corner with a Rorschach inkblot pattern of brown and yellow stains on its surface. A beat-up chest of drawers sits adjacent to the old grey metal bunk bed.

The odiferous body on the lower bunk stops snoring, rolls over, smacks his lips too many times and sits up.

"You the new guy?" He blinks at me. "Ken says you're crazy. I'm Jordan. Welcome to a psych ward posing as a recovery house. We're all fucking crazy here. You can take three of the drawers in that dresser. Just throw my stuff on the floor there. Where's your shit? Or are you like the rest of us here? Shitless. Hahaha."

Jordan rolls his legs over the side of his bunk and I identify the source of the stink — an open sore the size of my hand oozes on his left shin. I see exposed white bone. The infection is rancid and close to gangrenous.

He glances down and laughs. "Yeah, nice, eh? I had Gary pull out one of my surgery screws with a pair of pliers the other day. I'm going to go to the hospital, and they'll probably have to amputate."

Jordan loves the macabre attention his wound receives.

"For twenty years I was the boss of one of the biggest unions. Everywhere we went, everything high end. Whores — you name it, I had it. If anybody fucked around with the union back then ... we just took care of it. If you get my drift."

Jordan has that wild, unsettling psychopathic look in his eye. I've seen it before, when I worked in the correctional system in the early eighties with some of Canada's worst serial killers and violent sex offenders. Like most long-term crack addicts, what remain of Jordan's teeth are rotten and stained brown.

"I sure miss my girlfriend, Lucy," Jordan says. "She's a

good girl — twenty-two-year-old crack whore staying in my place Downtown Eastside. I'm a lucky old bastard. I can keep up with her all night long. All I need's my crack. I'd wear her out and go looking for her friend."

Hard to tell, but Jordan looks to be something between fifty-five and sixty-five.

"I'm on a methadone program," he tells me. "What medication are you on?" Most of the men here take some form of prescribed narcotic.

Ken returns to the dorm and laughs as he interrupts our conversation. "How do you like us so far, Crazy Mike?" He hands me an old sleeping bag and several ancient sheets.

"You should wash these," Ken says. "Good luck finding a pillow that doesn't smell like a sack of shit, though."

I don't want a pillow. I don't care.

I am about to share a bunk bed with a psychopathic, gangrenous heroin addict in a house run by a newly clean heroin addict in charge of administering prescription narcotics.

Biker Brad arrives with my briefcase. I stash it under my mattress in a precise position locked into my brain. If it is moved even the slightest, I will detect it.

For dinner we eat rice and boiled wieners with a bag of no-name frozen vegetables. Jordan approaches with my meds, the same Jordan fixated on pulling the screws out of his suppurating leg. He presents me with two pills — Keflex, which is an antibiotic, and an extra-strength Tylenol.

"Those aren't my meds," I say. That anyone has the gall to call a place like this a recovery home defies imagination. No one medically supervises drugs. No one performs any intake or assessment. No treatment plan is devised.

Later that evening, I lie on my back on the top bunk tracking the wolf spider that's navigating the spackled ceiling. Throughout the night, Psycho Jordan stares at me, silently.

He just stares and stares and stares.

When he notices me staring back, he averts his gaze. Two psychotics engaged in a macabre staring match. He scares the shit out of me. It's the dog that doesn't bark that's the most dangerous.

The next morning over coffee at the dining-room table, a young guy leans over to me.

"Jordan wants to kill you, Mike. He thinks you want to murder him in his sleep."

What remains of my clinical brain quickly deduces that Jordan measures high on the Psychopathy Checklist.

Grandiose estimation of self ... check.

Need for stimulation ... check.

Pathological lying ... check.

Cunning and manipulative ... check.

Lack of remorse or guilt ... check.

Parasitic lifestyle ... check.

Poor behavioural controls ... check.

Impulsivity ... check.

Failure to accept responsibility for his own actions ... check.

It's true I am paranoid, but my fear of Jordan is well founded. I become hyper-vigilant. If anyone is going to kill me, it's going to be *me*.

I later learn from the other guys that Ken steals other men's narcotics and methadone. He ingests anything he believes will give him a high.

Each morning, all of us attend AA meetings in Abbotsford. I hate the drive. The minivan is full of men smoking cigarettes. At the meetings, I stare at the walls, the ceiling, the floor. I can't speak because my scrambled brain won't allow me to articulate a thought.

At night, I attend the mandatory therapy group run by Neil, co-director of Mission Possible. He's working on his master's in eco-psychology. An impressive figure at over six foot five with a long, greying ponytail, he pulls up in his Mercedes.

Neil says he was once was a high-powered heroin and coke dealer who consumed most of his profits. In his therapy groups, he likes to tell stories of his numerous near-death overdoses and his conquests of women.

"They thought I was the best goddamn fuck they ever had or will ever have in their lives. I thought they were all cumbuckets anyway."

At meetings, Neil's style is to confront, cajole, belittle and berate.

"You're one crazy fuck," he tells one of the guys. "You're nothing but a fucking parasite. The only thing you care about is your next cigarette."

For men who've spent time in institutions or prisons, this authoritarian approach might actually work. But I doubt it. Compassion is hard to come by here.

One day, knowing I'm within earshot, I overhear him tell one of the men he's counselling, "Do you want me to tell you like it is, you fucked-up crackhead? Or would you rather I charge you a hundred bucks an hour and blow smoke up your ass, like some other fuckers around here do?"

I am that fucker to whom he is referring.

One day, as I sit depressed and suicidal, I hear the click of a camera. Neil stands above me. He's just snapped my picture.

"I'm going to send this to your kids. You sad fuck."

Hurtful, belittling behaviour is Neil's hallmark.

I watch him tear many other men apart and he seems to enjoy it.

Gary is a schizophrenic suffering from acute psychosis. Like so many schizophrenics, he does not have the capacity to care about personal hygiene. Nor does he have the cognitive capacity to process certain information. He is disoriented to place and time. He has difficulty connecting cause and effect. His capacity for abstract thought is limited. His concentration and ability to stay focused are almost non-existent. He cannot follow simple instructions.

One day, Neil has had enough of Gary. "Get out of here, you crazy fuck. You're nothing but a leach. Pack your plastic garbage bags and hit the road."

The next day, we see Gary panhandling in front of the local grocery store, homeless and stoned on crack.

Neil claims to be accessible by direct phone line from Mission Possible to his home an hour away. The phone is tucked into a small closet on a tiny table with a basic wooden chair. On the wall above is a sign with a number and the words "Direct Line to the Holy Spirit." The men call it constantly. The Holy Spirit returns your call if he considers you deserving. And that is rare.

A week after my arrival at Mission Possible, I'm not getting any better. I decide it's time to check out. Permanently. Maybe the third time will be lucky.

# 18

# CHECK OUT

I pull myself out of bed, get dressed and grab my beloved leather briefcase containing all my incriminating documents — police reports, charges, legal papers and my mountain of bills. I have not slept all night. I have a plan.

I go to the garage and retrieve a twenty-foot length of yellow plastic rope that I discovered in a pile of junk several days ago. Just like the rope Harold used. I stuff it into my briefcase and walk out of the house.

Two of the guys are sharing a smoke on the front porch.

Aussie gestures to my briefcase. "Hey, Crazy Mike, where you going? You got a business call or something?"

By now my obsession with my briefcase is an ongoing joke.

"Don't do it, Mike," Aussie says as I walk down the driveway.

"Just think about your boys, dude," says Cal. Cal and I know each other from Fresh Start. One night he revealed that when he was ten years old, he came home from school and discovered his father dead, hanging from the beams of their second-floor balcony. He was an alcoholic.

I carry on down the long gravel driveway, through the trees to the main road. I head to a large wooded area full of trails. I scouted through here the other day and identified a large tree somewhat hidden about twenty metres off the trail in the woods.

What has happened to my life? I love the woods. I wish I had a bottle.

Snapshots flip through my mind.

Me, at the beach, launching the boys over and over again into the water as they scream with glee. "Do it again, Dad, do it again!"

Making bows and arrows out of sticks and fishing line.

Swimming in the frigid water at Numb Nut Creek. That was the name I gave Paleface Creek, at the far end of Chilliwack Lake, where it flowed straight from the Cascade Mountain glaciers perched overhead. The boys' female cousins would blush and giggle every time we said "Numb Nut Creek."

I haven't alerted anyone to my plan. I've cried wolf too many times. I've lost count of the number of times I called my mother, my wife, my children, crying like a baby, telling them I was going to commit suicide. The first few calls sent them all spiralling into overdrive, marshalling resources to save my life. But after successive calls, when I actually didn't kill myself, they couldn't stand it anymore.

To love someone who is mentally ill or addicted or both is its own unique hell. That ongoing sense of fear and trepidation, not knowing if the person is going to die this time from driving drunk or from an overdose or will actually follow through on their myriad threats, is too much to bear. I remember how my mother would say, in the throes of desperation over my dad's repeated drunken binges, "It would be easier if he would just die."

I find my tree just off the main trail. I plan to bury my briefcase in the wet, mossy dirt under that log. The sun streams through the trees, lighting up the umbrella ferns. I smell the forest as it pumps oxygen into the air. It's a warm

April day, rare for this rainy time of the year in coastal British Columbia. The rainforest breathes, peaceful and silent. A sense of serenity descends. A memorable line of Chief Dan George's to Dustin Hoffman in *Little Big Man* comes to mind: "It is a good day to die."

I am reaching into my briefcase for the rope when I hear the sound of hooves on soft earth. Two people on horseback are slowly plodding my way. I do my best to look casual and inconspicuous, leather attaché case in hand.

I force a smile as they approach. The beautiful middle-aged woman and what must be her teenage daughter smile back astride majestic animals. They glance at each other and then, with identical wondering looks, size me up.

"Hello," says the mother. "It's a beautiful day to be alive, isn't it?"

I look around the woods. The trees stand tall and still. The sun's rays dance through the ferns and underbrush. The smell of hay and animal sweat steams off the horses. One nuzzles the other's glossy neck.

I haven't had a feeling like this in so long; at first I can't recognize it. Is it a sign from God? Keep going, Mike. Forget about one day at a time. Manage one moment at a time. Just this one beautiful moment.

After a short pause I reply, "Yes, it is."

As the horses and their riders saunter off around the bend in the trail, I stuff the death rope back into my case. Today is not a good day to die after all.

I emerge from the woods onto the paved country road. Briefcase in one hand, I thrust out my thumb. I will not go back to Mission Possible. A miasma hangs over that place.

An old blue GMC minivan approaches, slows down and stops. In an incredible stroke of bad luck, the driver is Ken from Mission Possible. He is the only one with a driver's licence. A cigarette droops from his lips. He glances deri-sively at my briefcase.

"Where you going, Crazy Mike. Business trip? Hahaha." He guffaws, and the rest of the van's occupants join in mirth-lessly through the smoke haze.

"Crazy Mike's on a business trip. He's hitchhiking to his next corporate meeting."

"He's in bad shape, Ken," Cal says from the back seat. "Don't you think he should go to the hospital?"

Ken agrees, nodding.

"The shrink needs to see a shrink."

Resigned, I get in the vehicle. Ken drives the ten minutes to the Langley hospital and orders me out of the van.

"We'll wait out here. Go in and don't fucking think about taking off."

Once again I sit with an admitting nurse, who escorts me to a side room.

"Wait here, Mr. Pond. The psychiatric nurse will see you shortly."

The clock reads 5:31 p.m. At 6:04, the psychiatric nurse walks in.

"Can you please give us a urine sample, Mr. Pond?" She hands me a specimen container.

After I hand it back to her, full, she begins the standard mental status exam.

"I'm not suicidal," I lie. Nope. Not psychotic. Not me.

As I stand waiting in the doorway, a patient in the bed across from me turns her head away and cries into her pillow.

She thinks I'm evil.

An old man to my left points at me and laughs.

He thinks I'm insane.

I sneak to the washroom down the hall. I look both ways, open the door quickly and step in.

"Hey, mister!" A woman sits on the toilet. Her four-year-old daughter plays in the sink beside her.

"Oh my God. I'm sorry." I run back to my exam room.

The woman, eyes big, scurries past me. She shields her daughter from the crazy old pervert who sneaks into ladies' washrooms.

The beds around me gradually empty. I am the only one who remains.

They're evacuating the ER. I'm under surveillance now.

The nurses check on me every fifteen minutes. Is that the police at the nurses' station?

The psychiatric nurse enters my room. "Mr. Pond, your lab work came back positive for benzodiazepines. Are you a drug addict?"

"No, I'm an alcoholic. I was given Ativan the other day at Peace Arch Hospital. Are the police here to arrest me?" I sweat. "They think I'm a sex offender. I went into the ladies' washroom by mistake. The door wasn't locked. A woman and her daughter were in there. I'm not a pedophile."

"It's okay, Mr. Pond. No one is here to arrest you. The psychiatrist will be here shortly to see you. Here, take this. It's olanzapine. It will help you relax."

"I don't want to take that. It's an antipsychotic. It'll knock me out."

"We can't give you a narcotic — doctor's orders. Please take this or we will have to give it to you by injection." How many times have I said those exact words to uncooperative patients? Without another word, I take the medication.

My head numbs and my eyes narrow. My arms and legs feel heavy, like wet wood. The olanzapine has kicked in. My thoughts wire together a bit. I can't stay here. They will lock me up.

Down at the nurses' desk, the police keep looking at me and laughing. They are here to trap me in a sting operation.

MICHAEL POND AND MAUREEN PALMER

But I'm too smart for them. Feigning nonchalance, I saunter into the patients' waiting room and pick up the phone. Hours have passed since Ken said he'd wait outside. He's gone home.

"Hey, Randy, can you come and get me?" I don't take my eyes off the police.

"What, Pond, are they releasing you?"

"Yes."

"We can't come and get you this time of the night."

"But it's only a ten-minute drive."

"I'm not coming to get you. You're on your own, Pond." He hangs up.

I bolt for the exit door and dart through the parked ambulances. The cold night air hits me like a slap. Shit! I forgot my briefcase. They'll read my documents and find me. I scramble back past the nursing station, grab the case and dash out down the long access road to hide in the trees.

It's cold. I wait and watch. No one comes after me.

# 19

# CRAZY MIKE WALKS AGAIN

I approach a plaza of small businesses and restaurants. I'm famished. I haven't eaten in two days. Several dumpsters on wheels huddle in the back lane. The green one: locked. The blue one: locked. The black one: open.

I rummage through layers of wet, smelly garbage and find a half-eaten Subway meatball sandwich. It's cold, the bread soggy with tomato sauce. It goes down in three chewless bites, bits of wrap included. Subway never tasted so good.

Somewhat satisfied, I head down the street and take a left on a gravel side road. I meander along in the rain and chill. The olanzapine keeps my thoughts settled, but I sense anxiety waiting in the wings.

What will I do? Where will I go? Whom can I contact? Nothing. Nowhere. No one.

I need to stash my briefcase. All the valuable legal documents, business statements, personal writings and bills have become too heavy to carry.

No, better not. Someone might find it.

A patrol car pulls up beside me and an officer gets out. His flashlight beam hurts my eyes as he approaches. He's very young, with a military haircut. He scans me up and down. I'm dressed in a blue polo shirt and jeans, my leather attaché in hand. "What are you doing out on the street this time of night," he demands.

I'm stumped for an answer. I shrug.

"Can I see your ID?"

"I'm sorry — I don't have any. I'm homeless."

"I know what homeless looks like, and you don't look the part." He points to my briefcase. "What do you have in there?"

"Just a bunch of personal papers and important legal documents."

"Really." Sarcasm oozes out of him. "Put it on the trunk and open it up."

I open it. The officer finger-shuffles through the stash of papers.

"Yeah. Wow. Looks like pretty important stuff." More sarcasm. He slides back into the patrol car. "Stay off the road or you're gonna get hit by a vehicle. It's dark on these streets. Take a bus to Surrey in the morning and go to Social Services."

I keep marching.

By now, the chill has crept into every one of my aging joints. I find a discarded sweatshirt in the ditch. It's filthy and stinks. I pull it over my head.

I spot a dilapidated shack with a caved-in roof nestled on the edge of a power cut-line. I crawl in through a smashed wooden door. The place reeks of piss and shit. Apparently I'm not the first homeless guy to find this little sanctuary. I pull a couple of splintery planks together, lay them on the ground and lie down with my briefcase full of secret treasure. Sleep comes in short, shivering snippets. Dear God, please let it be sunny tomorrow.

The sun rises and cracks through an opening in the wall at my feet. Thank you, God.

I gather myself up. My body aches. I step outside and find a tree to relieve myself.

I hit the streets again, scavenging for food under a bright, cold sun.

In a back lane, bins and bags are piled in small groups behind each home. It must be garbage day. I look both ways and lift lids to check inside each bin, careful not to get caught.

What's this? A small tray of macadamia-nut chocolate chunk cookies rewrapped in clear plastic — looks like something from a specialty bakery. Three whole untouched cookies left. Who would throw these out? What a find!

I wolf them down without taking a breath. I am so thirsty. Dry mouth — my brain flips through the *Compendium of Pharmaceuticals* and quickly makes the connection. It's a side effect of the olanzapine. A hose lies on the lawn. I sneak in through the open gate and turn the tap until a gentle stream flows silently out the end. Then I pee at the side of the garage. But I need to also have a bowel movement. I need to find a washroom.

No restaurants are open. Most establishments won't let homeless people use their facilities anyway. My stomach cramps and I sweat. I powerwalk the streets in search of ever-more-elusive public toilets.

Traffic is just beginning to move — early-morning commuters heading to work, oblivious to my predicament. I used to be just like them. I never had to think about how vital a private bathroom is to basic human dignity.

I find a Shell station on the next corner. The South Asian attendant stands behind a secure glass stall with a round metal speaker and a slider exchange tray. An array of cigarette cartons semicircles the wall behind him.

"Can I use your washroom?" I say into the metal speaker.

"Customers only." The young man speaks with a strong accent.

"I understand. But I really have to go."

"Sorry, sir. Customers only." He speaks mechanically. "We have not a public washroom."

"If I bought a chocolate bar, could I use your washroom?"

"Yes, sir." He nods.

"But I have no money. Please," I beg.

He squirms behind the glass. His fingers tap the counter. My eyes fix on his. They're dark brown, almost black, with heavy, long lashes. His eyebrows meet in the middle.

He slides the washroom key through the tray. It's attached by a thick chain to a piece of plastic the size of a laptop. No way I'm running off with this key ... although it sure might come in handy later in the day, or however long I homestead in the abandoned old shack.

"Thank you. I appreciate it." I snatch up the key and head to the washroom.

After my hard-earned use of the washroom and a quick cold-water face wash, I return the key. Able to concentrate somewhat, I look up at a calendar on the wall and realize I have no idea what day it is. "Could you tell me the date?" I ask.

"Tuesday, April fourteenth," he answers.

It hits me. I have to be in court tomorrow — in Penticton. That's a five-hour drive from here. My lawyer has delayed several times now, waiting for me to gain some sobriety time in rehab. I have thirty-four days behind me. Not long enough to impress any judge.

I find a lone pay phone in the parking lot of a plaza, in front of a Royal Bank. I press zero to get the operator.

"I'd like to make a collect call, please. 250-490-3434."

"Collect call from Michael Pond," the operator says after dialling the number. "Will you accept the charges?"

The phone receiver stinks of old saliva and bacteria. The last remnant of my old fastidious self is disgusted.

A female voice comes on the line. Jan, my lawyer's assistant, accepts the charges.

"Hello, Jan, it's Mike Pond. Is Matt there?"

"Yes he is, Mike. Just a minute. He wants to take your call."

A woman with a red setter walks by. The dog pauses and strains at the leash to sniff my rank self. Quite a wallop, I suspect, for his 200 million olfactory receptors.

"Hello, Mike," says Matt. "Where are you? We're due in court at nine thirty tomorrow."

"I'm on the streets again. I relapsed about a month ago. It's not good, Matt. I won't get a good report from the recovery house."

I fidget and shuffle from one leg to the other. My hips and lower back ache. A black Ford F150 rolls past. The young driver in a cowboy hat glances my way. My stomach growls.

"Listen, Mike," Matt says. "You have to get here now. I can't keep pushing this ahead. I thought you were doing well. You got a good job and a place to live."

"I was doing well, until a month ago."

"This is not good, Mike," he says. "Get here even if you have to hitchhike. I'll ask the court for another extension. And that's it. Be prepared to go straight to jail from court. Make sure you have a place to go to when you get out. Can you go back to that recovery house?"

"I don't have a suit. How can I go to court without a suit?"

"Who gives a shit about a goddamn suit? Just get here. I mean it."

"I saw you downtown last week, Matt. In front of the Hyatt."

"What? What the hell are you talking about?" Matt sounds confused.

"I saw you and your wife walking down Burrard Street."

"Oh my God. Yes, we were there for a weekend getaway at the Hyatt."

"I thought I was hallucinating. I was psychotic. I still am."

"Mike, I have to go now. Meet me in front of the court-house next Wednesday at nine o'clock. If you don't show, a warrant will be issued for your arrest. Can't your girlfriend drive you?"

"I'm not sure she's my girlfriend anymore. I haven't heard from Dana in weeks."

"Oh."

"Matt," I tell him, "I want my case waived to Surrey courts."

"When you waive, it's an automatic plea of guilty."

"Yeah. I know. I intend to plead guilty."

"I think that's best, Mike." The relief in his voice is audible. Not his problem anymore.

I thank him for all his help. He wishes me well.

Waiving my case to Surrey was Monk's advice. If the case is waived to the Lower Mainland, then Eli can go to court on my behalf and testify to my ongoing sobriety. I also want to save my boys and Rhonda the embarrassment of dealing with my drunk-driving record in my own hometown.

Matt is a good man. He agreed to represent both Dana and me pro bono. He managed to get her off the uttering threats charge. She had to agree to an anger management course and alcohol and drug counselling. I know I won't be so lucky. The thought of jail haunts me.

A bus approaches, headed for Surrey Central Station. The driver looks at me with my briefcase. "I'm sorry I have no money," I say.

"It's okay. Move to the back," the driver says.

I sit in the long back row against the window, my cheek pressed against the fog-cold glass.

The bus hisses to a stop in the notorious Whalley area of Surrey. What once used to be a respectable working-class neighbourhood has been overrun by addicts and dealers. Crazy Mike gets off and wanders amidst all the other homeless and mentally ill addicts. The shelters kick everyone out in the morning after breakfast.

"Hey, man, need meth?" a young man asks. Already they ply their trade.

I shake my head and keep walking without making eye contact, straight south on King George Highway. The olanzapine has completely worn off now.

Someone is going to kill me today. I will be baptized in the Holy Spirit. Is that John the Baptist? He is sent from heaven to kill me. No, it's Jordan the Psychopath from the Holy Mission Possible.

A horn honks behind me, and I jolt into reality and jump off the sidewalk onto the grass.

"Hey, Mike." It's Adam from Fresh Start and a couple of guys I don't know riding in his grey-blue '89 Honda Accord. It has rust all over the rear quarter panels and wheel wells. "Whatcha' doin' wanderin' the streets of Newton with your briefcase? You got an important business meeting or something? Get in. We'll give you a ride. Where ya headed?"

As I slide in the back seat, I say, "I don't know. I think I should go and admit myself to the psych ward at Surrey Memorial. I'm crazy, Adam."

"Well shit," Adam pulls the car away from the curb. "We don't need a psych ward to tell us that. We all know you're nuts, Crazy Mike. Let's go. We'll find you a shelter."

One of the guys gets on his smartphone and Googles men's shelters.

"Gateway House: full. The Front Room: no beds. Hyland House: full. Cloverdale House: yes, they have a bed."

"We'll drive you to Cloverdale, Mike," says Trevor. "You're not staying on the street. You wouldn't last a week here in Crackerville."

## 20

# CLOVERDALE
# HOUSE

We head east through Surrey and Langley and arrive in the outskirts of Cloverdale, a small rodeo town turned sprawling suburbia. The shelter is a small farmhouse refurbished to hold eight men. A pretty young woman greets me at the door. She is polite and respectful, probably a recent graduate from a local college or a social work student.

"Hello, Mr. Pond," she smiles. "My name is Ramita. I'm the supervisor this shift. Welcome to Cloverdale House. I'll show you around, then we'll do an intake assessment and life plan. We're a licensed facility subsidized by Fraser Health."

An assessment and life plan. Words I haven't heard in a long time.

A guy scrubs the toilet in one of the pristine bathrooms. A middle-aged woman chops fresh vegetables in the well-equipped kitchen. She wears rubber gloves. A couple of guys prepare a salad at the dining-room table. They both wear gloves.

Once again I'm bemused by the incongruities of my situation. Last night I wore a discarded sweatshirt stinking of vomit. Today everyone around me wears rubber gloves. This place is spotless.

The smell of roast chicken in the oven renders me incapable of thinking of anything but food.

At Mission Possible, dinner came after the five p.m. AA meeting. Being the new guy, it fell to me to make it. Twenty ravenous men would flood in, demanding dinner. Some would be especially hungry because they'd been out all day on construction sites. Randy, Mission Possible's director, known to the men as Rotten Randy, has a construction business on the side. Residents collect welfare or EI and work under the table for Rotten Randy and, I suspect, are underpaid.

But one can only get so creative with frozen wieners and potatoes, the only menu items available at Mission Possible. And in my state of heightened anxiety, to quote my dad, "I couldn't parboil shit for a beggar."

The guys mutinied.

"We're going to McDonald's," they yelled. "Can't eat any more of this shit. There's gotta be more than wieners to eat."

"Dunno what you fuckin' guys complain about," Rotten Randy said. "I buy groceries every week, and you eat them in the first three days. Lazy ungrateful sons of bitches. I've been running recovery houses for fifteen years. Never heard such a bunch of whiners in my life."

At Cloverdale House, a fellow about my age looks up, smiles warmly and says, "Hey, how are ya? My name's Gene. Dinner will be ready soon. You hungry?"

My reverie is broken. I don't comprehend. I stare blankly. It's been so long since anyone tried to engage me in a genuine and respectful fashion, I'm not sure he's talking to me.

"Hi, my name's Mike. Yeah, I am pretty hungry."

"Good. Get settled in, then fill your belly." He smiles. "The food is really good here."

"Come into the office, Mike," says Ramita. "This will take about an hour. Then you can put your stuff in your room." I follow Ramita into the little office.

A couple of guys laugh easily as they come in the back door, pull off their work boots and stand them neatly below the coat rack. Already, I feel anxiety wane.

"I need to ask you some questions. Standard intake information." Ramita writes on a clipboard.

"Okay," I nod, thinking ahead to that roast chicken.

"How did you end up on the streets?"

I offer Ramita a condensed version of my story, from my fall from grace in Penticton to down-and-out recovery houses in the Lower Mainland. Her huge brown eyes open wide. She listens intently.

"I just graduated from a social work program" she tells me. "This is my first job. You have quite a story, Mike."

"Yeah, I guess it is. It's not over yet."

"I need to ask you some questions about your mental status."

Uh, oh. Here we go. My stomach flutters — not from hunger this time.

"Have you ever tried to harm yourself?"

Ramita is compassionate and genuine. I see it in her eyes. "Yes, Ramita, I have. I tried to hang myself, drown myself and jump out of a moving vehicle. I have nothing to live for."

She averts her eyes for a second. She doesn't want to ask the next question. But she does.

"Do you have suicidal thoughts now?" Her gentle demeanour disarms me.

"Yes, I do."

"I need to call Car 87, Mike. We don't have the resources here to help you. They're a police and psychiatric nurse partnership that respond to mental health emergencies. You need professional help. We're just a shelter."

"I'll be okay," I protest. "I don't need to see a psychiatric nurse. I *am* a psychiatric nurse."

"I have to do this, Mike. It's the law. I'm concerned for your safety. They will come here and do an assessment. Just go and try to relax in your room."

Why did I tell Ramita I was suicidal? Why can't I keep my mouth shut? Why do I keep sabotaging myself? Having worked in mental health for three decades, I know the stigma associated with being certified. I still hold on to a shred of hope that someday I'll work again.

The RCMP patrol car pulls up. A young constable and a rotund woman in her late fifties step out and approach the house. She's an old warhorse from the mental institution days — I can tell from the self-assuredness of her walk. She's done this a million times.

I hear Ramita fill them in outside my door — everything, including my status as a health care professional.

"He says he wants to kill himself. He's agitated and very anxious."

The psych nurse comes into my room and pulls up a chair while the young constable stands in the doorway, his hands clasped in front like a soccer player protecting his privates for a penalty shot. He's ready if I bolt.

"Hello, Mike. My name is Belinda. I'm a mental health nurse, and this is my partner, Ron. We came to do an assessment and help you."

I don't want to prolong this. The outcome is inevitable now.

"I have suicidal thoughts," I explain, "but I don't have a plan at the moment."

"But you have made attempts in the past?" Belinda asks.

"Yes, I have."

I know her next line verbatim.

"You are not safe, Mike. They can't keep you here.

They're not equipped for this sort of thing. Are you on medication?"

"Yes, Celexa and trazodone, but I haven't been taking it. I don't trust the recovery house to give me my correct meds."

"Mike, as a professional, you of all people know you have to take your medication. You will never get better. What's in the briefcase?"

"All my important documents."

"Ah, I see. Where are your belongings?"

"At the recovery house. I don't care about any of it."

"Let's go. We're taking you back there. But first we're stopping at the pharmacy to refill your prescription. You're going to start taking your medication now. If you don't, we'll take you to the hospital. Got it?"

I know that the place I'm standing in right now offers the best possible chance for real recovery. But I've blown it. Back to Mission Possible.

Belinda, the constable and I walk into the local pharmacy. Belinda tells the pharmacist my situation. The pharmacist enters my information into the computer and nods. "Yes, he is prescribed, Celexa and trazodone. I'll fill it immediately. The costs are covered by Social Services and Housing."

Once filled, Belinda hands me the two bottles. "Take these right now. And keep taking them as prescribed," she orders.

We get in the cruiser and head southeast to Langley, destination Mission Possible.

"You were a psych nurse in the Okanagan," Belinda says. She names a colleague who works up there. "We graduated together in 1971. She moved there twenty-five years ago. A community mental health nurse."

I slip into rational thought for a moment. I surprise myself with my clear-mindedness. I think I surprise Belinda, too.

"Yes, I worked with her in the early nineties. We started

the provincial pilot project for Mental Health Urgent Response Services in partnership with the RCMP. It was the beginning of this program that you guys do now. I was the program manager." Back then it would never have occurred to me I'd need the services of the very program I helped create.

"Do you still have your nursing licence?" she asks.

"It's being reviewed right now."

"I don't think you should be nursing. You're not competent to practise. I'm going to report you to the College." She nods. Well, take a number and stand in line.

The blue and white police cruiser glides up the treed lane to the house. Two days after my failed suicide attempt, after two nights of wandering, I'm back at Mission Possible.

I'm cursed.

It's sunny and warm. Several of the guys are smoking on the front porch, and they bolt when they see the cop car. Crushing their cigarettes in the gravel, Ken and Jordan approach the vehicle with caution.

"Looks like you found Crazy Mike," says Ken. "I used to be an auxiliary police in Chilliwack. Before I became a heroin addict, that is."

The constable says, "Can we have a look around the place? A little tour of the facility."

Jordan and Ken exchange queasy glances. I spot Cal peeking out the small bathroom window. I hear the toilet flush. The guys are getting rid of their stuff. The house is on red alert.

As Ken tours the guests around the house, all the men have mysteriously disappeared. The place is deadly quiet.

Belinda looks around the messy dorm. "This place is a disaster. Do you guys not have any health standards? Is this place licensed? Who's in charge here?"

"I am," says Ken. "I'm the house manager."

"How long have you been clean and sober?" Belinda asks.

"Two months," Ken says.

"Oh my God! Who's responsible for administering the medication?"

"I am." Ken says.

As expected, Belinda disapproves. "You're an addict! I'm going to report this place to the Health Authority. Here, Mike." She hands me my medications. "Make sure you take your meds every day. We're going to follow up on this place."

Ken throws me a sideways sneer as we follow the constable and Belinda out the door to the patrol car. Ken and Jordan wave and smile sardonically. I hang my head.

"What are you thinking, Pond?" Ken spits on the driveway. "Bringing the fucking cops here. That's all we need is the fucking authorities roaming around here."

"I'm on parole," says Jordan. "They could've hauled my ass to jail."

Ken immediately gets on his cellphone. "Hello, Neil? He's back. He showed up with the cops. They were checking the house out. Okay. See you in a bit." He flips his phone closed. "Neil will be here in a couple of hours. He's not happy."

A couple of hours later, Neil, the house therapist, arrives. I step out the front door. There he is, in studied repose, leaning against his black Mercedes. A cold smile breaks his handsome face.

"Well, well, Dr. Pond," Neil smirks. "You spineless piece of shit. I thought you wanted to off yourself. No balls, eh? Come on, let's go. I'll drive you to the Port Mann Bridge right now myself. We'll stop at Canadian Tire and pick up some rope. Let's go. Let's fuckin' go."

I look him directly in the eye, do an about-face and walk directly back into the house. Fuck you, Neil.

"What the fuck do you think you're doing, Pond? Coming back here with the cops," scowls Psycho Jordan.

Slowly the guys slink back, emerging from their respective hiding holes, like rodents after the cat has departed.

"We're really worried about you, Mike," says Cal. "We don't want anyone offing themselves here, man. That scares the shit out of everybody."

"I'm here on probation, for fuck sakes. I coulda been breached," a new guy says.

I take the stairs down to the dorm. Neil's cruel goading has managed to accomplish what nothing else has. It's yanked me out of my suicidal spiral. I often think that it was pride that took me down. Too proud to admit I'm powerless over alcohol, I'd drunk so much my illness had spun so out of control, I'm losing my mind. But I know psychosis ebbs and flows. I've observed my own clients, deep in its grasp, display unpredictable yet perfect lucidity. Right now I'm lucid and prideful and thinking there's no way the old Mike Pond would put up with this bullshit.

I am a professional, and I will not let that bastard get the better of me. I'm better than him. I will get sane and sober just to prove it. I haul out my briefcase, plop it on the bed and, click-click, it flips open. An unopened letter from the Fraser Health Authority sits on top. After I relapsed, this letter was sent to Fresh Start. It's been forwarded to Mission Possible, and only now do I have the courage to open it.

*Fraser Health Authority*

*Mr. Michael Pond,*

*Please contact Ms. Colleen Slater, Fraser Health Authority Occupational Health Nurse, as soon as possible to begin the process of assessment to make a determination regarding your possible return to work.*

*Yours truly,*

*Robert Lyons*

*Human Resources Manager*

*Fraser Health Authority*

I take a sharp breath. I can't believe it. I'd only been on the job a few days before I blew it, showing up drunk. They actually might give me a second chance. Gripped by five parts anxiety and one part hope, I call.

"Hello, Ms. Slater? This is Michael Pond."

"Yes, Michael," she says. "I've been trying to reach you. The people at the number on your personnel file said they didn't know your whereabouts."

Fucking Fresh Start.

"I'd like to set up a meeting with you as soon as possible," she continues. "Since you disclosed your alcoholism to your supervisor, we want to develop a gradual return-to-work plan. The College of Psychiatric Nurses has already made medical monitoring a condition of maintaining your licence; Fraser Health will now be part of that monitoring. We have received a report from Dr. Acres, and he has provided us with recommendations for you. I'll set up a meeting with HR, the union rep, the College of Psych Nurses and management for next Monday at nine. Are you able to make it?"

My tongue catches on the back of my front teeth.

"Yes. Yes. I will be there. Thank you so much."

I march straight to my bunk and scribble out my own treatment plan to present at the meeting.

*Will abstain from alcohol and all non-medically prescribed substances.*

*Will be medically monitored by an addictions specialist.*

*Will provide random urine samples as directed.*

*Will attend three AA meetings per week.*

*Will attend addictions counselling with a qualified therapist.*

I smile to myself. I've written plans just like these when my clients needed them.

Mere hours ago, I was fixated on offing myself. Now I'm fixated on showing Neil and Rotten Randy and Ken, the bastards, that I will make it. For the first time in a long time, I'm aware of feeling hungry.

I walk up the stairs into the kitchen. The new guy stands at the stove, boiling rice. Again.

"There's nothing to fucking eat here," he grumbles. "Randy hasn't bought groceries in weeks. Nobody can reach him. Ken says he's in Vegas on our rent money."

I fling open the cupboards in search of anything to augment our carb-rich diet. The cupboards are largely bare, save for a fifty-pound bag of pancake flour, a commercial restaurant-sized box of spaghetti and remnants of a five-gallon pail of rancid, rock-hard peanut butter. And bread. Lots and lots and lots of donated day-old bread. Randy tests the theory that man cannot live on bread alone.

*Clinical Notes — Mental Status Exam:*

*Appearance: Patient appears slightly dishevelled, unshaven and gaunt. Behaviour: Psychomotor retardation. Speech: Slow and hesitant. Mood: Depressed and anxious. Perceptions: congruent with no evidence of psychosis. Content of thought: no suicidal intent. No plan. Motivated to regain employment. Affect: Wide range, angry. Insight: fair, developing a better understanding of illness. Judgment: good. Global Assessment of Functioning: 60/100 — Moderate symptoms.*

Psycho Jordan still stares all night convinced I want to kill him in his sleep. The rancid odour of serious infection wafts from his leg. He gets up in the middle of the night to change the dressing, clogged with pus and caked blood. He uses old plastic wrap and tape that he keeps stuffed under his pillow. No sterile technique here.

"The fucking hospital won't cut it off, so I'm going to amputate the fucker myself," he says, half to himself, half to me.

I drift off into the best sleep I've had for six months without booze as an anaesthetic. The trazodone finally works. Or is it a certain sense of peace of mind? Or is it both?

Each morning I force myself to go for a long walk. It's quiet in rural Langley. The early-morning sun turns mist to dew on freshly cut grass. A rooster crows in the distance. The odd farm truck rolls by with a load of hay. A hobby farmer in a Lexus wears a business suit and heads into the city to begin a day of work.

Back at Mission Possible, a half-dozen sets of old Nautilus fitness machines, donated by a local gym, sit in the garage. I push myself to work out every day. I read my AA Big Book every day too, and meditate on its principles and slogans:

*Easy Does It*

*Live and Let Live*

*But for the Grace of God*

*First Things First*

*One Day at a Time*

*Let Go and Let God*

I memorize entire passages. I learn the Prayer of St. Francis by heart.

I hate the meetings but attend every day. The Elis, Randys and Neils are asked to share at every meeting and speak of honesty, love, compassion and acceptance. But life in Fresh Start and Mission Possible is about shame, judgment, recrimination and intolerance. The dissonance rankles.

When I last visited Dr. Acres, he told me I needed $600 to begin medical monitoring. With the possibility now of my job continuing at Fraser Health, I've got to get someone in my family to lend me the money for medical monitoring. I'm forced to ask, yet again, for money.

I call my dad's wife, Christel.

We've shared a few conversations recently that make me hopeful. She told me my dad had been waking up in the middle of the night, crying out my name. Dad has been sober now for coming up on twenty years.

She picks up.

"Christel, I need your help just this one time, please. I need just enough money to get my medical monitoring started so I can work again as a nurse. Six hundred dollars."

"Yes, Mike," she says, "I will help you. But we can't ever do this again. If you drink again, this will never happen again."

Going out on a limb for me is way out of Christel's comfort zone. Her stolid German upbringing taught her self-reliance.

"Thank you," I stammer. "I appreciate it. I won't disappoint you."

Christel wires me the money. Another break.

Through May and June, I stick religiously to my own personal program.

Concentration improves and I can finally put a pen to paper. I return to work on my Step 4 — "Make a searching and fearless moral inventory of yourself." I write page after page, day after day.

*The times I got drunk on camping trips, during holidays and at hockey tournaments.*

*The times I staggered about our hometown falling-down drunk in a state of oblivion.*

*The embarrassment and shame I caused my family.*

*The countless times I didn't show up at work and was not there for my clients in their times of desperate need.*

*The times I showed up but was so hungover and sick I was useless.*

*The time I missed my niece's wedding in Manitoba. She had given me the honour of being the MC. I got drunk instead and didn't show.*

*The times I drank and drove and put innocent people at risk.*

*The times I took money from the business and my family to buy booze.*

*The many breaches of trust and damaged relationships with family and friends.*

*The times I stole to support my addiction.*

*The thousands of times I lied to my wife and my sons about my drinking.*

*The times I made my mother cry.*

*The times I made the boys' mother cry.*

I survey the list. If I ever end up getting my life together, I'll have to spend the rest of it making amends.

Others in the house notice my new focus and energy.

"What the hell's got into you, Crazy Mike?"

"You on a mission impossible? Hahaha."

"Crazy Mike's turned into Professor Pond?"

*Clinical Notes — Mental Status Exam:*

*Appearance: Patient clean-shaven, well groomed, good eye contact. Speech clear and articulate. Mood: Positive, rates it 6.5/10. Affect: bright. Concentration: good. Perceptions: No distortions in perceptions of reality. Content of Thought: Mood-congruent, goal-focused. No evidence of psychosis. Insight and Judgment: good. Global Assessment of Functioning: 65/100 — Slight impairment, good functioning.*

The Celexa is reaching therapeutic levels. Celexa is a selective serotonin reuptake inhibitor, or SSRI. It changes the balance of serotonin, which helps brain cells send and receive chemical messages more effectively. It elevates mood. It improves concentration. It diminishes obsessive thinking. It reduces anxiety. It works.

The comments keep coming. "Who the fuck are you? You look ten years younger these days."

"Hey, man, you're looking good," says Wayne. "You're fun to be around now."

Carey smiles. "Hey, Pond. I didn't know you could laugh."

As sanity returns, awareness of just how bad things are at Mission Possible sinks in.

Jim, a young heroin addict, worries. "Ken is watering down my methadone," he says. "I know he's taking it. Why do you think he sleeps so much?"

"Yeah, man," Colin pipes in. "My dosage seems weaker too. He's dipping into it. Lazy fucker sleeps all day."

"I found bags of potato chips, beef jerky and chocolate bars hidden in his room. The rest of us eat rice and pancakes every day," says Wayne.

"Randy drives around in that big Mercedes," says Colin. "He hasn't been around for days. I hear he's in Vegas again."

That things could actually get any worse at Mission Possible is a bit of a mindboggler. But the expectation that I can recover in a place where the inmates are in charge of the asylum makes me resolute: I must return to work at a place where mental health treatment is credible and compassionate. I will get my job back.

# 21

# A SECOND CHANCE

Early Monday morning, the sun streams in my bedroom window. Just recently graduated from my dungeon dorm to an upstairs bedroom with four beds, I'm not used to the brightness. On this beautiful June day, I will meet with the Fraser Health Authority. It's been two months since I wandered the streets of Surrey and Langley.

Nervous and excited, I rush downstairs to a makeshift barber's shop set up in the kitchen. I sit up tall, propped on a stack of couch cushions on a kitchen chair. A warm towel nestles on my neck as Aaron, a young guy of about nineteen and a new resident of Mission Possible, gives me a standard jailhouse haircut. A buzz cut with electric clippers from Canadian Tire with a number-two attachment; then he lathers my neck with Gillette blue gel. He finishes the job off with a Fusion 5 blade.

I gaze with satisfaction at my reflection in the mirror.

"There," says Aaron. "You look like a cop for sure now. Or an old-time gangster. Or both. Hahaha." He hands me a pair of brand-new black cords. He's a small guy like me.

Wayne offers me one of his brand-name golf shirts. It's a white lightweight Nike with a Tiger Woods logo.

"That's a hundred-and-fifty-dollar shirt, Mike." Wayne grins.

Aaron says, "Here's my dress shoes. Florsheims my uncle gave me. He's a bigwig downtown lawyer."

The men stand back and admire their handiwork.

"Man, you look great, Pond!" Wayne claps. The guys all nod in agreement.

For the first time in a long time, I feel proud of myself. Then a wave of nostalgia washes over me. I miss the guy I used to be. I grieve his loss. That's followed by a rush of gratitude, for the circle of support around me. In the midst of their own struggles, these guys who have not much have given it all to me.

"Hey, Mike, Ken won't get up," Rob says. "I knocked and knocked on his door. He took his usual shitload of everyone's meds last night. He's out cold. How are you going to get to your meeting?"

Wayne pipes up. "I'll drive you. I'll go in there and grab the keys."

"No, you better not. You'll get kicked out," says Rob.

"I don't give a shit," says Wayne. "I hate this fucking place."

Wayne disappears into Ken's room. Ken's snores echo throughout the house.

Wayne emerges. "Let's go," he says. "I've got the keys. There's no way you're missing this meeting, Mike."

Rob, Wayne and I head to Langley Memorial Hospital, the hospital where just seven weeks ago, I had a psychotic break. This is where the occupational health nurse has her office. In a hospital environment, an occupational health nurse helps employees who've suffered health setbacks return to work. I've suffered quite the setback.

This is my ticket out of Mission Possible. This is getting my life back. This meeting is vital to my recovery. I sweat.

It is 8:20. A woman waits for me at the reception desk. "Hello, Michael." She shakes my hand. "My name's Colleen

Slater. I'm the OHN for Fraser Health Authority. I'm your case manager. I'm pleased to meet you."

"Hello, Colleen. It's nice to meet you."

In a warm but business-like manner, she explains the process.

"You'll meet with your union representative first on your own. She'll fill you in on your rights as an employee. That meeting is strictly confidential. At nine o'clock we'll all meet as a group. That meeting is also confidential; however, the proceedings of that meeting will be documented and kept in your employee file."

Now Maureen Ashfield, the union rep, joins us. Her warm smile and the empathy in her eyes quell my rising anxiety. "Hello, Michael. Let's go into this other office for a private meeting," she says.

She immediately lays out the union strategy. "Fraser Health claims you didn't meet your probationary period. We say you have. It's June tenth. As of June second, you have been an employee of Fraser Health for three months. They say you went off sick after your first week and have not worked since. We say they put you on a medical leave. They did not try to contact you. We say no. We think we will win that argument."

I can't believe what I'm hearing. The Health Sciences Association — of which I haven't been a member for two decades, is fighting for me. By turns, I'm shocked, surprised, skeptical and grateful.

"Michael," says Maureen, "you have rights as an employee through the collective agreement. Furthermore, you have a medical illness. Dr. Acres diagnosed you with severe chronic alcoholism. You're going to get help. It looks like Fraser Health will not pay for treatment. Nor will they pay for Dr. Acres' assessment. However, they *will* pay for the ongoing monitoring. In any event, we will keep fighting for you."

Colleen knocks on the door and peeks in. "We're ready."

I step into the meeting room with Maureen. Several people watch me. I recognize Kay, my manager. She doesn't look up. She writes furiously in a notebook. Everyone holds a copy of Dr. Acres' report. I sit down. The HR representative hands me a copy and another one-page document on Fraser Health letterhead.

Everyone smiles. Finally, I breathe.

"Michael," explains the HR rep. "This is the agreement the Review Committee has drawn up. It identifies all the terms and conditions. It is a gradual return to work, beginning with quarter-time, and over a one-month period you will be back to full-time. This agreement is for two years. You must meet all the conditions. Breach of any of the conditions will result in disciplinary action and possible termination."

Hands shaking, I scan the terms.

1. Remain abstinent from alcohol and all addictive substances.
2. Undergo medical monitoring by Dr. Acres on a biweekly basis.
3. Provide laboratory samples as ordered by Dr. Acres and/or the management of Fraser Health Authority for a period of two years from the date of this document.
4. Provide random chain of custody urine samples within 24 hours of notice from Dr. Acres' office.
5. Attend at least three AA meetings per week.
6. Ongoing regular meetings with an AA sponsor.
7. Regular biweekly meetings with the Fraser Health Authority Occupational Health Nurse.

I read them all and read them all again. They're very similar to what I proposed for myself not so long ago. I take a deep breath and read them all yet again. The trapezius muscles in my neck and back finally release. Tears flood my eyes. Very slowly, I look up. Everyone stares at me with expectation. A knot of emotion chokes me. I take another deep breath.

I nod and whisper, "Thank you."

Kay says, "It's good to have you back, Mike. You can start back on the unit next Monday."

Six copies of the agreement circle the table, and each representative signs. My not-so-reliable left hand tremors a squiggly version of my signature on each copy. I brace my hands on the table, push my chair back, stand up straighter than I have in a long time and shake everyone's hand — firmly. Thank you. Thank you. Thank you.

I leave the office, my head high, body erect, and walk purposefully through the long halls of the hospital and out the main exit doors, the mid-morning sun's rays warm and welcoming on my face.

Where's the van? Where's Rob? I scan the parking lot. Nowhere.

I survey the main waiting area. No Rob or Wayne. I find a pay phone and call the house.

Rob answers. "Ken called me back to the house soon after we got to the hospital. He was really pissed off, Mike. He made me bring the van back. Now he's gone with it. He said you could find your own fucking way back."

It's over ten miles back to the house. I don't care. I'm so elated that I'm getting another chance. I walk. I stick out my thumb, but no one picks me up. Buoyed by the outcome of my meeting, I walk and walk. It takes just over three hours to make it back to Mission Possible.

As I walk up the wooded winding lane to the house, I spot Ken standing on the front porch smoking with Psycho Jordan. He wears his usual baggy black sweatpants. A crumpled wrapper from an Oh Henry, my favourite chocolate bar, rests by his foot.

"How was your morning stroll, Pond?" he says with a smoky snort.

Beside him, Jordan snickers into his grimy, nicotine-stained fingers. His nails are filthy. I can almost smell the oozing infection on his leg.

"It was very nice, Ken," I say. "It's a beautiful day. I return to work on Monday."

"Well, congratufuckinglations. And how are you going to get to work, Dr. Pond? I'm sure as hell not going to get up at five a.m. to drive you," he sneers.

"I'll find a way." I walk through the house and see most of the guys hanging out in the sun in the backyard, their shirts off, smoking and laughing. I smell fresh-cut grass.

Rob smiles. "You got it, didn't you? I can tell by your face."

A round of genuine congratulations erupts from the gathered men.

"I start Monday morning," I tell them. "Getting there is the big challenge. The closest bus service is in White Rock. That's a twenty-five-minute drive and then forty minutes on the bus to Surrey Memorial. I wish I had my bicycle."

"Don't worry, Mike," says Rob. "We'll get you there. Fuck Ken."

The week passes like cold molasses in January. Ken ignores me most of the time. Sunday night, the guys all pool their money and give me just over twenty dollars, money to bribe Ken to give us the van. The gesture makes me cry.

I can't sleep from the anticipation of working back at the hospital. How will the staff react to me? How many know what happened? What will they say? How will they treat me? Can I do the job?

Thank God for the College of Psych Nurses. Thank God

for the union. Thank God for Dr. Acres. Thank God for the Fraser Health Authority.

I wake up in the dark. The numerals on Rob's clock radio glow red from the far corner on his chest of drawers. If I squint just right and strain my neck far enough without falling out of the bunk, I can read the time. It's 3:16. The minutes click forward. Time just doesn't move fast enough sometimes.

Finally, 5:15. The Sony blasts Aerosmith's "Janie's Got a Gun." It's still dark outside. Rob quits Steven Tyler's wailing to curses from the other men who share our room.

"Shut that fucking thing off."

"Son of a bitch."

"I hate fucking Aerosmith."

"Let's go, Mike," Rob whispers. "It's time for the old guy to go to work."

I shower and shave. I wear the same clothes that I wore to the meeting last Monday. Everything freshly laundered and ironed. I look good. I feel great.

The old GMC van fires up. The gaping rust hole in the muffler rattles and bangs in the silent night air. The tall cedars stand still and watch and listen. The pebble gravel grinds under my feet as I climb in and slam the door shut. A dog barks from somewhere down the hill.

Twenty-three minutes later we pull up to the White Rock Central bus loop. As I grab the door handle, Rob says, "Hey, we got the van. I'm gonna drive you all the way."

"Thanks, Rob. I guess it's okay. I don't know how I'm going to get there every day. I've got to get money for bus fare. I only have enough to get back to White Rock today."

"We'll figure something out. One day at a time. Let's just get you there today."

We arrive at the hospital's back entrance at 6:25 — thirty-five minutes early. "I'm going in," I say. "I'll meet you guys at the Fiver and get a ride back to the house."

The Fiver is the daily five-o'clock AA meeting at the Masonic Hall in White Rock. It's a large open meeting that all the men from Fresh Start attend every day. Eli makes it mandatory. The guys from Mission Possible have recently begun attending too.

It's quiet at the hospital's south entrance. All the action happens at the north main lobby and the ER. I know — I've been there, as both patient and staff. The security guard welcomes me with a warm, tired smile.

As I walk down the first long corridor, my footsteps echo off the pale blue walls. At the end I notice the familiar sign: Adolescent Psychiatric Unit. The APU.

The unit is secure. I lost my ID pass card that opens the door. I look in the tiny Plexiglas window and see Faith sitting at the nursing station's main computer monitor. I tap on the window. No response. A little harder and Faith looks up, nods and presses the buzzer to let me in.

I move tentatively toward the counter, unsure of what to say or do as I move around the desk and into the back room of the nursing station.

"Hi, Faith," I say.

She turns away without a word and puts her belongings into her backpack. She looks tired. Faith was running the shift the night I was sent home drunk, back in March. She was very nice to me prior to that. Asked me copious questions about my private practice in Penticton.

"I'm tired," Faith says. "Ray is in the TV room with a psychotic kid who's been up all night. The meds are counted. You just have to sign. I'm going home. Goodbye." Silence as the metal door clunks shut behind her.

Ray emerges from the TV lounge with a young Middle Eastern boy in his early teens dressed in brown hospital pyjamas. Ray is a youth care counsellor in his mid-forties who wears a perpetual snow-white smile, but not this morning. He's been expecting me. He too was on shift the night I went home drunk.

"Let's go, Amar," says Ray. "I'll take you to your room. We have to lock your door to keep you safe. Don't make any noise. Everyone is sleeping."

I accompany them to Room 1 without being asked. I know the routine. Room 1 locks with a large deadbolt. It is used for kids who are unpredictable and considered a danger to themselves or others. A camera in an upper corner of the room feeds to a colour monitor in the nursing station. Anyone in there is on constant observation.

Ray bolts the door shut to the boy's protests. Amar beats on the locked door several times then stops. Ray still hasn't acknowledged me. I follow him silently back to the nursing station as he scoots a wheeled office chair up to the monitor. He focuses in and observes Amar move about like a silent shadow in the big box with a bed. It always reminds me of security camera shots from the 7-Eleven or the bank.

The unit access door buzzes open. Janice, a veteran nurse in her mid-fifties, hobbles in, her knees already aching from too many years on the job. The last time I talked to her she was waiting for elective surgery. She's twenty-one minutes early for her seven-o'clock shift.

"Hello, Mike. You're back to work again, eh?"

"Yes, Janice. It's good to be back."

She nods sideways in Ray's direction and, just low enough not to be heard, whispers, "Some aren't so sure."

"Yeah, I can see that."

"I understand you're on a gradual return to work," she says to me. "Management says you have to have a buddy assigned to you for the first month until you're full-time again."

"Yeah, that's the plan."

"Looks like I'm your girl today. I'll put you on meds with Mark."

Janice likes to be the boss even when she isn't the boss.

Ignoring my presence, Ray debriefs her. "You're working with Mark and Jim. Busy day. All three psychiatrists are in for rounds. Three sets of parents are in this afternoon for case conferences. Beverly has ECT this morning at seven thirty. She's all prepped to go. Allison cut her wrists when she was out on pass over the weekend. She's out cold on PRN meds. She's stitched and bandaged up. Be sure to check her dressings. Calvin's blood sugars are out of whack. He keeps sneaking food. Kelson keeps spreading shit all over his room. He'll need a bath this morning. The RCMP brought Jess in yesterday. He assaulted his mother. He needs his injection the minute he wakes up. Security is alerted. He punched one of the security guards when we secluded him last night. He spit right in Kate's face when she gave him his injection. You have three discharges and two new admissions due at any time. Typical uneventful day at APU, eh? Everything else is on the shift report. And oh yeah, a bunch of summary reports are due today. Have fun! I'm gone." Ray avoids eye contact, grabs his backpack, shuffles past me and heads out the door.

Janice opens the shift report on the computer and reads each patient's synopsis, as well as a long list of tasks and duties. "Looks like I'm going to be a busy woman today," she sighs, and pulls out a clipboard for the staff. She writes furiously on the duties sheet, intent on organizing everyone's day.

"I know Mark's in charge," she says, "but he can't delegate a damn thing. Too young and too damn nice. How are you doing, Mike? You just started in March and then you were gone."

I pause, think the question through for a moment and say, "I'm okay. I had to take a medical leave. It's good to be back working."

A pregnant pause hangs in the air. I don't fill it.

"Hmmmmm. I see. I hope things are okay."

The door buzzes open. Mark, a nurse, and Jim, a child care counsellor, arrive next.

"Good morning, Mike," Mark says.

"Hi, Mike. Welcome back," Jim says.

"Hi, Jim, Mark. Thanks."

The team is outwardly cordial. But they must resent me. I know *I* would. They fear I can't be trusted. And that's a big concern when dealing with the erratic, unpredictable and often violent behaviour of young psychiatric patients. They await my next screw-up.

We all grab coffees and pull a tight circle of chairs in the tiny staff room.

I haven't worked in an institutional setting since 1989 — over twenty years ago. I was a thirty-five-year-old supervisor in a unit very similar to this one. The technology has advanced so much. The medication has changed significantly. Policies and procedures are different. My brain is older, and alcohol abuse has taken its toll. This team won't cut me any slack. Nor should they.

Can I measure up? Can I pull off the role of psychiatric nurse, a real functioning person? I'm scared it's just a matter of time until I'm discovered to be an incompetent fuck-up.

The briefing barely over, the morning erupts into organized chaos.

Janice barks, "Mark, get security down here. I have to give Jess his injection. He's pulled out all his stitches. I need Mark and Jim to assist. You come as a backup, Mike."

Backup is hard to screw up. Jess is suffering from a drug-induced psychosis, something for which I now have special empathy. The seclusion room is pale blue, with a bare plastic mattress on the floor. A grey blanket lies bunched by the mattress. Janice peeks in the tiny window. Fourteen-year-old Jess curls up in a fetal position, picking at the open cuts on both his wrists. He has pulled out his sutures. The brown- and red-stained bandages pile in the corner. Finger-smears of blood cover the walls.

Jess screams. "Let me out of here. I want out! Let me out!"

Three security guards arrive in uniform, pulling on vinyl gloves. They are silent and ready. We all put on gloves and gowns.

"I can't stand it!" howls Jess. "Let me out. Please let me out."

Janice, matter-of-fact, says, "Jess, we are coming in with security. We have to clean your cuts and give you your medication. Please get up and stand in the far corner facing us."

One guard unlocks the metal door with two heavy dead bolts. The smell smacks us. A pile of feces sits in the corner at the centre of a pool of urine. Mark's face contorts in disgust. "Man, that's nasty! Jim, grab some towels and soap," he says.

Jess stands up naked, covered in blood and shit. Both of his wrists bleed. Blood covers his mouth and chin. "No! Don't hurt me! Don't hurt me!"

"We are not going to hurt you, Jess," says Janice. "We are here to help you. We are going to take care of your cuts and clean you up."

Two security guards flank Janice. We're behind. A guard grips the sheet coiled in his hands. Janice holds a small plastic tray with two syringes.

Jess' eyes are wide and wild, his naked, sinewy body taut. His fists curl tightly at his sides. "No," he says. "You are not giving me a needle." He thrusts his chest and face deep into Janice's and spits in her face.

In an instant, the younger guard jumps in front of Janice and takes Jess down with a chokehold. The boy's arms and legs flail. The other guard jumps in and hogties his legs with the coiled sheet. Then they flip him over onto his stomach.

"Easy, guys," says Mark. "Not so rough. It's okay, Jess. We're here to help you. Try to relax."

Janice quickly and efficiently injects two syringes of medication, loxapine and lorazepam, into Jess' elusive squirming buttocks. Loxapine is an antipsychotic. Lorazepam cuts the anxiety. I know they work. I've been on them myself.

"No. No. No," he wails.

Within minutes the lorazepam begins to take effect. Jess' squirming eases and his body settles. Jim nods at security and they ease their grip and, in slow motion, back out of the room.

Mark removes the sheet from Jess' legs.

"That's it. Just relax. You're okay. You're okay," Mark whispers as he gently cleans the blood and muck from the boy's arms and body with warm, soapy towels. Jim wipes up the urine and feces in the room with disinfectant and places clean pyjamas on the mattress.

As everyone backs out of the room, Janice says, "Just let the medication take effect, Jess, and we'll come back in a little while and put fresh bandages on those wounds."

"Good job, everybody," says Jim. "Are you okay, Janice?"

"Oh yeah, I'm okay. Just another day at APU."

Janice is okay, but I'm stunned. I've been so long gone from any kind of professional interaction with acutely psychotic patients, I no longer believe I have the capacity to stay cool under pressure like Janice and Jim and Mark.

I try to be unobtrusive. "Just move through the day and try to do no damage," I repeat to myself, like a mantra. The psychiatrists arrive one by one. The social worker arrives in his Birkenstocks. The psychologist. The occupational therapist. The recreational therapist. The unit teacher and her assistant. The unit clerk. The janitor. The lab tech arrives to take blood and urine samples. I get swept up in the steady flow of life on an adolescent psychiatric unit. I don't have time to think about the dynamics of my return until it's time to update the patients' charts.

*The patient demonstrates psychotic ...*

*The youth has poor appetite and ...*

*The patient refused to ...*

Why can I not write? Why won't my brain function?

In frustration and embarrassment, I turn to Mark, whose fingers fly over the keyboard. He stops and looks at me. "You okay, Mike?"

"If I tell you about my patients, Mark, would you mind writing it for me? Then I'll sign the progress note."

I fully expect rejection and putdown, because that's the normal response to everything in recovery houses.

Mark sees the anxiety in my eyes. I see empathy in his.

"Sure, Mike. No problem."

Breathe now.

Three o'clock. The shift ends. Only when I interacted with the children was the anxiety almost bearable. I got through it. I didn't kill anyone.

I walk off the unit and trudge to the bus stop, aware of an odd sense of accomplishment. You made it, Crazy Mike. You made it through your first day of gradual return to work.

I step out the back entrance of the hospital onto 94th Avenue, into the bright sunshine. Dozens of teenagers stream from the high school across the highway. They mill about eating chocolate-dipped cones and Dilly Bars. Largely carefree, the story of their lives yet to be written. I wish them all happy endings.

A survey of the surroundings tells my own story. To my left, Creekside Withdrawal Management Centre, where I spent twelve days detoxing. To my right, the Phoenix Centre, where I spent five weeks in treatment. I see men smoke and laugh at the back entrance. I should be there. But I broke the rules, went AWOL with Dana and snuck in booze.

Today I pay my full fare when the bus arrives, two dollars and fifty cents. I don't know how I'll pay tomorrow.

I get off at the final stop on the corner of 152nd and North Bluff Road. I walk down the hill, south toward the beach. The city bustles with locals and tourists. It's that time of year. I can smell the ocean mixed with french-fry grease and hot new pavement. The city workers wind up their day, load construction tools onto a paving truck.

I arrive at the Masonic Hall. The Fiver meets here 365 days of the year. I'm excited to "share" when the chair calls on me, because finally I've got good news to report. I've got my job back. I'm sober. After a round of congratulations, the meeting breaks up and an old-timer sidles up to me. "Way to go, Mike," says Sam. "Let's go for a coffee?"

"Yeah, Sam, that would be great."

We pull up to the Tim's on 152nd Street. It's packed with the supper crowd, and a long line weaves its way out the door. We wait and I vent.

"I can't stay at Mission Possible any longer, Sam," I say. "I have to find a place closer to work." I tear a huge bite from my whole-grain sandwich, with the wrap peeled back just enough to expose a wad of chicken salad with lettuce and tomato. I know I should chew slowly to savour every bite, but I'm ravenous. Next, I shovel the piping hot chili back and wash it all down with a gulp of hot, creamy, sweet double-double coffee.

Sam smiles in silent bemusement.

"Do you remember young Max, the welder?" He sips his black coffee. "He sobered up at the Fresh Start a few years ago. He rents a small house on Russell Avenue just behind Peace Arch Hospital. I'm his sponsor. He's looking for a roommate. Somebody in the program. You'd be perfect."

My heart leaps out of my chest. A chunk of chicken falls out of my gaping mouth. I can't believe it. Freedom.

"I think you could move in right away," Sam continues. "The guy who shares with him is getting married. He just moved in with his fiancée."

"How will I cover the rent? I have thirty-eight cents to my name. There's one week left in June, and I don't get paid until next Friday." My mind races. I do the math. About $480, before tax and deductions — that's about three hundred bucks. My heart plummets. But wait, I have one more welfare cheque coming to me this Wednesday! I have to get that cheque before they forward it to Mission Possible, and I have to get a cellphone because Dr. Acres' office will phone any day for my first piss test. I can't rely on Ken to take any messages if I'm not around or at work. Fuck!

"Take it easy, Mike," Sam says. "I'll call Max right now. I'm sure he'll figure something out for you." Sam dials a number on his cellphone and fills Max in.

A pause.

"Yeah, I think he's good for it ... Yeah, he's right here. I'll let you talk to him."

I take the phone.

"Sam says you're doing great," says Max. "Keep working the program. I'm twenty-four and I'll be four years sober in September. One day at a time. So I'm looking for a roommate. I'm away on the pipeline here in Northern Alberta one to two months, then back home for a week or two. You'll have the place to yourself most of the time. Sam can take you over to have a look. It works out to about thirteen hundred a month including utilities and cable. That's six-fifty each."

"That's great, Max. I can give you three hundred next Friday and the rest in the middle of July."

"Don't worry about it, Mike. I don't get back till about then. The rent is paid up till the end of July. You're a professional with a great job, and I know you're good for it. This is awesome."

"Thank you so much, Max. You don't know how much this means to me. I'll talk to you later." I press End on the phone, look at Sam and grin.

"I'll take you up to have a look at it." Sam gets up, jangling his car keys. "Max told me where the key is hidden."

We drive to a tiny two-bedroom bungalow built in the fifties. Peeling paint and an overgrown lawn greet us. Like me, she's past her prime. Inside, the hardwood floor is scratched and well worn, the furniture old and sparse.

"It's perfect, Sam." My eyes sweep around the house as I imagine living here. "And just a ten-minute walk to the bus stop directly to work." My brain calculates rapid-fire now.

All recovery houses have an agreement with Social Services and Housing to have the monthly cheques signed over to the director of the facility. I have to intercept next month's welfare cheque before Randy picks it up on Wednesday. No one can know I'm leaving. Rob is the only one I trust.

When I get back to Mission Possible, Rob and I sit out back behind the shed while he enjoys a smoke.

"I found a place in White Rock. I can move in right away," I say.

"Holy shit, Mike. That's great. Who with?"

"Young Max the welder. He's about your age, Rob."

"Yeah, I know him. He's a good guy. He's been sober quite

a while. He's never around, though. Works up north all the time. You'll be there by yourself."

"I know. It's great."

Rob's brow furrows. "I don't know, Mike. You think you're ready to be living alone? You're only sober a few months. How about Two-Finger Ted's sober house? They're looking for a fourth roommate."

"Nah, I'm sick of living with a bunch of maniacs. Especially you. I'm ready to be on my own. I'm beyond ready. My only concern is getting out of here and snagging my welfare cheque before Randy gets his hands on it."

"Good point. Good luck. He's gonna be pissed off."

"I don't give a shit."

That night I borrow Wayne's cellphone and call my son Brennan. "I've got a dilemma, Bren. I have the choice of moving into a house with this young guy named Max. Except he'll be away working up north seventy-five percent of the time. So mostly I'll be by myself. Or I can move into a sober house with three other guys who attend AA and are active in the program."

Brennan — my middle child. Always contrary. My biggest challenge in parenting. Ironically, now he's the only one in the family who still communicates with me. In my downward spiral, many who loved me blocked my tortured calls, but never Brennan.

"I don't think you're ready to live on your own yet, Dad." Brennan sounds hesitant. "Maybe at some point down the road, but not yet."

I know he's right. But I crave peace.

"Okay, son," I say, "I'll think about it. Either way, I have to get out of this place."

"I get that, Dad. But I don't think you should live alone yet. You don't do well when you're alone. You're a people person."

I hear the worry and concern in his voice. I hear the fear.

Live with Max? Move into the sober house? The autonomy. The independence. The freedom. The risk. I don't trust my own mind. Rob and Brennan are right. I should move into the sober house.

I'm moving in with Max.

# 22

# PAY DAY

I may have a full paycheque and a new home in two weeks, but today I don't have two nickels to rub together. No bus fare to return to work tomorrow. And I have to pay off Ken for use of the van.

"Rob. Let's spend the day collecting bottles and cans."

All morning and most of the afternoon, Rob and I walk the ditches of rural South Langley hauling large, heavy plastic garbage bags. We wade into ankle-deep mud to retrieve half-buried Bud and Coors Light and Kokanee cans and the odd pop can from the culverts. Our treasure is mostly beer cans, obviously thrown from moving vehicles. The irony is not lost on me.

While we're at it, we pick up all manner of filth and litter. People on bikes and cars slow down to see what we're doing.

"Hey, that's awesome. I drive by every day and the garbage is getting disgusting."

"I've got a box of bottles and cans in my garage. You guys can have them."

"Thanks, man. A lot more people should be out here doing this."

By noon, both our bags are jammed and we have to go back to the house to get new ones. Far from the humiliating experience I assumed this would be, it's exhilarating.

By four o'clock we have four bags full of every can and bottle imaginable.

The grand total: $84.40. Twenty dollars protection money goes to Ken.

Rob and I split the remaining $64.40. That's $32.20 each — bus fare to get to work for a week and half till I get paid.

Sleep comes more easily tonight but doesn't last. Wayne's clock radio reads 3:47 a.m. I tiptoe to retrieve a one-pound bag of Starbucks coffee hidden in a gym bag under Wayne's bed. It's our secret. I brew a small pot and savour every hot sip.

"Hey, is there any more of that Starbucks left, old-timer?" A sleepy Rob goes to the pot and pours himself a mug. He drinks. "Damn. I wish we had cream and sugar. Fucking Randy. I know Ken has some stashed in his room. Fucking lazy prick."

I shower, shave and slip into Wayne's freshly laundered golf shirt. Rob's got Ken's car keys, this time with his consent because we paid him off. We climb into the van and drive in companionable silence. The yellow-orange sun climbs behind us, lighting the trees and hills ahead. Finally, Rob speaks.

"I was thinking about it all last night, Mike. I don't think you're ready yet to live on your own."

"Rob. I've made up my mind. I'm moving into Max's house."

The silence continues all the way into White Rock, where Rob drops me off at the bus stop. "Have a good day, buddy," he says. "See ya at the Fiver."

I walk onto the unit three minutes before the seven-o'clock shift starts. In unison, Jim, Janice and Mark say "good morning" then return to the business at hand, morning reports. No warmth, just politeness.

Janice says, "Mike, we put you on meds. You might as well get started. You're partnered up with Mark again today."

The med room. I gulp. If I screw up here, something really bad could happen.

Each time I encounter a medication I'm not familiar with, I pull out the *Compendium of Pharmaceuticals* and read the dosages, action and adverse effects. Most are new-generation antidepressants, mood stabilizers and antipsychotics: Zyprexa, Seroquel, Risperdal. My hands shake as I portion the pills and liquids into tiny paper and plastic containers.

Mark peeks in. "How's it going? Do you need anything?"

"No, I think I'm okay. I'll call you if I need to."

Putting pills into their appropriate paper cups isn't the problem. That hasn't changed in twenty years. Logging the meds in the computer and ordering more — I don't know what the hell I'm doing.

Bloodwork orders, X-ray requisitions, admissions, all done on computer. Mark, Kate and Sarb see me struggle and offer to help, but they go so fast I can't follow. So much of this stuff is now second nature to them. Over the afternoon, I see their frustration levels rise. They can't get their own work done because they have to teach grade nine word-processing to a fifty-five-year-old man.

On the bus ride back to White Rock, I get off at the Newton Exchange and stride into the social services office. It's Welfare Wednesday. I bypass the long lineup of people waiting for their cheques and go directly to the counter. "Hi, my name is Michael Pond. I have an appointment with Susan." Susan is the young woman who worked her supervisors to get my six months of hardship welfare.

"Hello, Michael. You're looking well," Susan says when we sit down in her office.

"Thank you. I've started work again at Surrey Memorial. I don't get my first paycheque till next Friday. I'm moving out of the recovery house as soon as possible, but I need my social assistance cheque to make a deposit on my new place."

"Congratulations." Susan smiles. "It's good to see you're getting back on your feet. So this will be your last cheque from us. Good luck."

"Thanks, Susan. I don't mean this in a bad way, but I'm glad to see the last of you."

When I arrive in White Rock, I go to the bank and cash my cheque. Six hundred and ten precious dollars. Today I keep it all. It's been a long time since I've had that amount of cash in my hands. I finger through the twenties, making sure Queen Elizabeth looks the same on each one, and then marvel at the Bill Reid Aboriginal creation memorialized on the back.

At the Fiver, Sam introduces me to Keith, Max's soon-to-be-departing roommate.

"Hi, Mike." He shakes my hand. "I hear you're moving into the place. It's a nice little house. You'll like it." He hands me the keys.

"I can give you six hundred bucks, Keith," I say. "That's all I have. I can settle the rest next Friday when I get paid."

"That's fine. Sam says you're a good guy."

I count out each bill for Keith, until I only have a lonely ten left. Dour Sir John A. Macdonald perpetually frowns. He thinks I'm making a mistake, too.

With what's left of the bottle and can money, I now have $38.45 to get me through the next nine days. After the Fiver, Ken drives us all back to Mission Possible. The entire ride I stare out the window, ignoring everyone. I'm out of that damn place tomorrow. I can hardly believe it.

I pack my belongings. Again. I cannot even count the moves I've made in the last four years.

After five hours of solid sleep, I awake refreshed and raring to go at 4:11 a.m.

"Let's go, old man. You're movin' on up," laughs Rob.

"Shut up," I scold. "The last thing I need is to have Randy find out I'm ditching this place."

I get Rob to drive by the little rundown house on Russell Avenue on the way to the bus stop. In the break of dawn's light, behold: a mansion. After work I'll stop at the Safeway and buy a few things. Maybe make a couple of barbecued burgers with melted cheddar cheese and sit on the back deck. Enjoy a quiet meal in the sun.

Work is unusually quiet. It's Friday, and many of the kids will go home on a weekend pass. That seems to have a sedating effect on everyone, staff included.

"Is Mike Pond here?" I hear a familiar male voice down the hall. "I need to see Mike Pond."

I know that voice, but it shouldn't be here. It belongs to Dangerous Doug, my old roommate from Fresh Start. I step out of the meeting room and there he is, his thick bulk hanging over the desk at the empty nursing station. How the hell did he get into a secured unit? He must have followed the food cart or the janitor in. What the hell is he doing here? My head swivels to see if anyone is watching.

Doug looks at me — excited at first to have found me, then ashamed. "Mike, Mike, I had to come. I have something to tell you."

As I near him, I can see and smell he is dead drunk.

"I need to make amends, man. I told your girlfriend that you were dead. I told her you offed yourself. I'm so sorry, man. Please forgive me, man. I was drunk when I did that. I'm so sorry, man." He was drunk then, and he's drunk now. As quickly as I can, I absolve him. I've got to get him off the unit before anyone sees us.

"That's okay, Doug, I'm not dead. I'm fine. It's okay, but you need to leave." I shuffle him out the door, as he chants over and over, "I'm so sorry, man. I need to make amends."

I return to the nursing station, where Janice sits, looking down the hall at Doug. "Who was that?"

"Just some guy from the streets I ran into. Must have followed me in to work," I shrug.

On the bus ride home, I fidget and squirm and plan. I'll do a couple of loads of laundry. I'll make my dinner on the barbecue. I'll watch what I want on the forty-seven-inch flat-screen TV. I'll sleep in that beautiful king-size bed in Max's room. There won't be a snore to be heard, except mine. Perfect peace.

When I get off the bus, I cruise into the Safeway. It's cool, bordering on cold. I pick up a head of iceberg lettuce, a vine-ripened tomato, extra-strong Canadian cheddar, three crusty kaiser buns from the fresh-baked bulk bin, butter, milk and finally the hamburger — lean Alberta Angus beef. I noticed yesterday all the necessities in the fridge and cupboards at Max's house. Ketchup, mustard, relish, salt, pepper and Kraft's original barbecue sauce.

I can't stop smiling as I pay for my groceries with cash. The summer sun shines brightly as I bounce down the Johnston Avenue hill toward the ocean, the bulging plastic grocery bag bumping playfully against my calf. I saunter around the corner of Pacific Avenue and pass the RCMP station where I spent the night in the drunk tank just six months ago, on one of the coldest winter nights on record.

I spot Rob standing outside the Masonic Hall having a smoke, waiting for the Fiver to start, chatting up two young girls. He hurries over to me.

"Hey, Mike. Rotten Randy's really fuckin' mad. He heard you left the house and that you scooped your cheque. He's here looking for you. And oh yeah, that doctor's office called the house. The woman said ... let me think. Oh yeah, it was something like ... it's time to go to the lab."

The wind drops out of my sail.

"Shit." My shoulders droop. "I have to go for my piss test. I have twenty-four hours." It's my first random urine test for Dr. Acres, and it's the last thing on my mind. I gave his office the house client phone number. Rob and I had made a pact. We'd meet every day at the Fiver. When the call comes in to go to the lab, Rob would let me know. If all goes as planned, I'll be able to afford a cellphone by the end of the month.

Just then, Rotten Randy rounds the corner of the building. Quick-footed, smoke in hand, head strained forward like a big vulture intent on his prey. He jabs his cigarette at me.

"Where the fuck is your rent money, Pond? You didn't give a month's notice. I want it right now!"

"I gave it to my new landlord. I'm moving into a house here in White Rock tonight."

"That money is mine." Randy's cigarette punctuates his words. "You're not ready to live on your own. You'll be drunk within the month. You're so full of shit, Pond."

"It's done, Randy. There are lots of guys waiting to get into the house. You'll get your rent money."

Randy pulls a big drag off his cigarette and blows the smoke in my face. It's acrid and sweet. His snakeskin cowboy boots grind in the gravel as he about-faces and slithers off, smoke cloud trailing behind him.

"I'll get my money, Pond," he says. "One way or the other."

After the meeting, I walk the eight and a half blocks to the little white house on Russell Avenue. Randy's spiteful prediction still unsettles me.

Fuck him. Fuck them all. I will stay sober this time.

# 23

# PISS TEST

I light up the gas barbecue on the back deck. It's 6:57 in the evening, and the sun is still high in the southwest. After the chaos of Mission Possible, the peace and quiet is a little unnerving.

In less than nine minutes, I devour both burgers, washed down by a half-litre of Coke. I can't believe I'm free of that hole and sitting in my own place. Max's music selection is superb — for someone who's fifty-four, not twenty-four. The Rolling Stones' *Exile on Main Street*; Led Zeppelin I, II, III and IV; the Allman Brothers' *At Fillmore East*. Ah, here's the one! Paul Simon's *Graceland*, the best album of all time.

I insert the disc and "Diamonds on the Souls of Her Shoes" fills the little house and echoes out the door into the back deck and yard. I lie on the plastic moulded lawn chair, intertwine my fingers behind my head and close my eyes.

"Well, hello there, Mr. Pond. You look very handsome lying there all by yourself in the sun."

My eyes snap open. Dana moves slowly and sensuously toward me in a pair of khaki shorts and a white sleeveless cotton top, red flip-flops flip-flopping on her red-toenailed feet. She slides her sunglasses to the tip of her nose, lowers her chin and peers straight into my eyes. "I've missed you, Mr. Pond. Your little recovery-house friend, Wayne, told me your new address. He's such a sweet young man. Kind of cute, too."

Dana leans down and plants a vodka-flavoured kiss on my lips. "It looks like you're stepping up in the world again, Mr. Pond. You couldn't have gone much lower, that's for sure." She looks around the yard.

I want a drink. I reach for my diet Coke and take a big, unfulfilling swig.

Dana takes my hand and we go into the bedroom, lay on Max's king-size bed and have sex. It's frenetic and brief at first, then unhurried and lasting till close to midnight. Only now that she's here do I allow myself to admit how much I've missed her.

I wish the night would never end. I wish we could just curl up together and go to sleep, wake up and make love again, make coffee and go to work like real people, not like drunks. Already the act of leaving has begun. She dresses and pins her hair wordlessly in the mirror.

How many times have I discovered those pins hiding in the sheets? How many times have I watched her leave in the middle of the night? How many times have I wondered where she goes after she leaves me?

I think back to the first months of our relationship when we were both trying to stay sober. That was another Dana — bright, funny, engaging and mesmerizing, the perfect balm for my loneliness. We went on road trips to Whistler and the Kootenays; stayed in romantic B & B's. Shot pool. Played tennis. Slow danced. Made love.

That Dana doesn't come around anymore. Her alcoholism has advanced considerably since we first started seeing each other. Her life now seesaws between increasingly shorter periods of regret-fuelled sobriety and devastatingly destructive benders. I want to be with her. I hate myself for wanting to be with her. I have met my perfect match.

"I have to go, Mr. Pond," Dana says to her reflection.

"Are you still seeing Stu?" I ask. Stu is Dana's new giant biker-boyfriend.

"We won't be talking about any of that now, will we, Mr. Pond?" She shifts and poses in the mirror. "Let's not ruin a beautiful evening."

I lean on my elbow in bed and watch her smooth her shirt and shorts and pick up her purse.

"It's the Gay Pride Parade soon," she says. "Why don't we make a date to go and then head down to the beach at English Bay?" She gives me a fleeting peck, wipes the red lipstick from my cheek and slips out into the warm July night.

I race to the front door to watch her pull out.

The black top of the Miata comes up as Jon Bon Jovi yowls "You Give Love a Bad Name." She's an eighties girl, and she doesn't want to mess her hair.

My mood sinks as I watch the Miata peel away down Russell Avenue. I have to go to Surrey in the morning to give my urine sample. I want a drink and I want it badly. But I won't. I can't. It's after midnight and thank you, Lord, the liquor store is closed.

When I wake up Saturday morning, the clock radio by Max's bed reads 6:41. I haven't peed since Dana left last night, and my bladder is going to burst. Typically, I get up in the night at least once and then I go again when I wake up. I have to hold my urine until I can give a sample. If I can't give a sample, I will have to wait at the lab for up to an hour to make another attempt. If I can't give a sample it will count as a positive test ... which is a fail. If I can't give a sample, I'm done.

Across from the bus loop, an old street guy with a full shopping cart takes a leak against the wall of the community centre. That could be me. That *was* me. An even worse realization: that could be me again. It would be so easy to slip. What seems an eternity later, I get on the next bus and get off at King George and 96th Street. I shuffle to the lab. Thank God, there are only a few people waiting. I take a ticket and sit down to wait.

The lab tech behind the counter calls out, "Number eleven."

I look at my ticket. Fifteen. Shit. Breathe, Mike, breathe.

A few minutes later, "Number twelve."

Still later, "Number thirteen."

Even later, "Number fourteen."

"Number fifteen." Finally. Thank you, Lord.

Close to tears, I squeeze my knees together, clench my jaw, and waddle to the counter and hiss, "My name's Michael Pond. I'm here for a drug-screen urinalysis."

The lab tech purses her lips and says, "Can I please have your health card and driver's licence?"

I pull my British Columbia ID card out of my pocket. "I don't have a driver's licence. I don't have a health card. My number should be on your file. Dr. David Acres has ordered this monitoring."

The tech's large brown eyes narrow into a hint of a scowl as she takes my ID. "Do you have a requisition?"

"No, I don't. They didn't give me one. This is my first sample. Listen, I really have to go. Can we hurry this up?"

"I'm sorry." She sniffs. "I can't do the procedure without a requisition. And I need your health card."

"Look, I got the call yesterday from Dr. Acres' office. I have to give this sample today. Can you call his office to get a requisition?"

"It's Saturday, sir. I'm sure his office is closed." She blinks at me.

"Please. I have to do this today."

"I understand that, sir, but I need the requisition. Number sixteen."

"You can't do this!"

An older lab tech overhears us and slides over to the desk with an empathetic glance at me.

"Let me have a look at Mr. Pond's file." She pecks on the keyboard, waits a few seconds. "Ah, there it is. Yes, Mr. Pond. I see Dr. Acres' order here, on your Fraser Health file. It's a chain-of-custody procedure. [Chain-of-custody means the process is safe-guarded against anyone cheating.] Please have a seat and someone will be right with you."

"Thank you very much," I say, almost peeing my pants with relief. The anticipation of finally going is unbearable. I pace the waiting room, breathing deeply as if in labour.

A young lab tech calls out into the room, "Michael Pond."

"Yes. That's me." The waiting room is full now and everyone watches the show.

"Follow me and empty all your pockets and put the contents into this." The tech hands me a plastic Ziploc bag. I put my wallet, a few coins, the house key and a flat white rock I found at the beach months ago. A girl on the street called it a worry stone. It has been rubbed shiny smooth.

"Is that it?" She stares suspiciously at me as she wiggles her fingers into vinyl gloves. She's done this a thousand times and has good reason to be suspicious. Hardcore addicts are notoriously inventive when it comes to passing drug screens.

Other patients perched on chairs giving blood samples watch the process.

"Now use that disinfectant and wash your hands thoroughly."

I follow her instructions. The tepid water on my hands makes me want to pee beyond imagination. A warm dribble leaks into my jeans.

The tech opens a small white box, lifts out a urine sample bottle in a tiny plastic bag and draws a line at the three-quarter mark with a black Sharpie.

"Fill it at least to this line. Any less and it's unacceptable as a valid sample. Go into that washroom. Do not turn on the faucet, and do not flush the toilet. I'll be here waiting. When you come out, give it to me directly, then wash your hands again."

I go into the washroom. The toilet lid and flush handle are taped unceremoniously with brown packing tape. So are the sink handles and faucet. The toilet bowl is full of dark blue disinfectant.

My hands shake with anticipation as I hold the tiny bottle at the end of my penis. I'm afraid I will blow the bottle out of my fingers with the coming torrent. Here it comes. I squeeze the bottle tight. Urine sprays and splashes everywhere, and within 2.75 seconds I overflow the bottle. I gingerly set it on the small counter and continue to pee into the deep blue bowl for an eternity. I close my eyes, lift my head to the gods and moan in utter relief.

The lab tech takes my dripping sample and checks the bathroom for any monkey business. She unfolds a multiple-copy form.

"Initial here, here, here, and sign and date here." She wipes off the sample bottle and seals it with red tape, drops it in the plastic bag, stuffs it in the little box, places the white copy of the form in the box, closes the box and seals it with more red tape. She scrawls her initials on the tape and instructs me to do the same.

She hands me the yellow copy of the form, and I'm done.

I jump on the bus and enjoy a relieved ride back to White Rock. I did it. I gave my first chain-of-custody sample. Odds are I have a two- to three-week reprieve until the next one.

I spend a good part of the day watching TV and listening to music, stuff non-drunks do. Mid-afternoon, I explore the house and the tiny attached garage. The garage is full of Max's work tools and welding equipment. I spot an electric mower with a hundred feet of cord by the door. I plug it in and press the red start button, and the blade whines. For the next hour and a half, I cut the scraggly, dandelion-infested lawn, front and back. It feels good to work. When finished, I take another hot shower, get dressed and walk to the Fiver. I must attend the Fiver every day. This is my program. And this time, it will stick.

# 24

# BACK TO WORK, WEEK TWO

Monday, July 13, 2009: the start of the second week of my gradual return to work. Three full days, one more than last week.

The unit is full with ten kids aged twelve to eighteen, all suffering severe bouts of mental illness. All very sick, otherwise they wouldn't be here. Major depressive episode, anxiety disorder, bipolar disorder, obsessive compulsive disorder, schizophrenia, substance-induced psychotic disorder. As I walk past fourteen-year-old Amar, who is struggling with a major depressive episode with psychosis, I flip up my shirt and say, "Hey, Amar, ever see a grandpa's six-pack?" The sight of my scrawny grey-haired chest and wrinkled washboard abs cracks him up. It cracks up the staff, too.

Mark, Sharon and I escort several of the kids on an outing to the inlet at Moody Park. The mood is light; the kids tease one another, and for just a little while on this hot summer day, they're just regular kids.

Amar abruptly breaks the spell. He stops walking and stares at a man who appears to also be of Middle Eastern descent. Amar goes berserk. He screams, "Go away go away go away!" and bolts across the park, looking back and shrieking at the man, who is thankfully oblivious. Amar is delusional. He flees toward the water, to the pier. He stops at the end, turns and screams, "Leave me alone leave me alone leave me alone! I'm going to jump."

He watches me, his fear palpable. He thinks I'll hurt him.

Agitated and excited, the other kids run toward the pier too. They're so tightly wound that if one comes undone, they all do.

"Mark," I shout. "Gather up the other kids and keep them at the picnic table. Too many of us on the pier and he'll jump."

I advance up the pier. Calmly. Quietly. Slowly.

"Amar, I am going to help you. I won't touch you. The man is gone. You are safe. I am going to walk with you. I won't touch you, and we'll talk about what's going on. That man is gone, you are okay, you are safe. You are safe. You are safe."

Slowly I edge ever closer to him, talking in a soft, soothing tone. As I get closer, I see his body begin to relax. We walk back to the van. I sit with him and engage him in conversation. He is floridly psychotic.

The afternoon hijacked, we gather up all the kids and return to the unit. Amar rests in the quiet room. I suggest we debrief with the kids and staff. One by one, each kid reveals what it was like to watch Amar go berserk and how it made them feel. Tension drains from the room.

"Mike, it's really great to work with someone who knows what he's doing," Mark says.

"Why aren't you working full-time?" asks Kate. "You're needed here."

I work intensely with each kid, every day. It's my job to make them laugh, support them, give them hope. Get them to buy into their recovery, to believe that they can get better.

When I'm in the Adolescent Psychiatric Unit, I rarely think of myself.

The rest of the week passes uneventfully. Each small task or chore, the day-in, day-out ordinary stuff of life, brings enormous satisfaction. Folding my laundry. Cooking a steak. Taking a hot, steamy shower and staying in there until I emerge like a shrunken prune.

In an odd way, I miss the guys at Mission Possible, like Rob and Wayne. I see them at the Fiver, and we go out for coffee sometimes after the meeting.

Friday, payday. I have a penny and a quarter in my shorts pocket. As I walk onto the unit, Stephanie, the unit clerk, hands out envelopes to the staff.

"Here you go, Mr. Michael James Pond. That is your full name, is it not? May I see a valid driver's licence please?" She laughs. She doesn't realize just how funny that is.

"Thank you, Steph." I rip open the envelope and inadvertently tear a small corner off the cheque inside. Damn. Relax, Mike, relax.

I read it. And read it again. Then read it once more.

*Fraser Health Authority.*

*Payable to: Michael James Pond.*

*One thousand two hundred and thirteen dollars and seventy-two cents.*

I inhale with an airy whistle. Holy shit. I stuff the cheque into my backpack. Zip it up tight.

Come back a minute later, unzip it and make sure the cheque is still in there. Then take it out. Read it again. Make sure the numbers and letters haven't magically disappeared.

*Fraser Health Authority.*

*Payable to: Michael James Pond.*
*One thousand two hundred and thirteen dollars and seventy-two cents.*

I fold it in half and slip it into my back pocket. Throughout the day, I duck into the bathroom and pull it out of my back pocket. Read and reread. I pat my pocket all day to ensure it's still there.

*Clinical Notes — Mental Status Exam:*
*Appearance and Behaviour: Well-nourished, physically fit. Excellent personal hygiene. Dressed neat, clean and casual. Walks erect and purposeful with good eye contact. Speech: Clear and articulate. Mood: Positive, congruent. Affect: Bright, smiles spontaneously. Perception: No distortions in perception of reality. Thought Processes and Content: No evidence of psychosis. Displays some obsessive tendencies. Oriented to all three spheres. Insight and Judgment: Good. Global Assessment of Functioning: 75/100 — Good.*

All day, I fantasize about what to do with that paycheque. Pay next month's rent and the rest of the damage deposit. Buy groceries, real fruits and vegetables. Shop for new clothes and runners. Get a cellphone.

When I emerge from the bathroom for probably the eleventh time, Mark says, "What's the matter, Pond? Do you have the shits or something? You've been in the can all day."

"Yeah, I'm not feeling well. I've got a bug or something."

"A woman named Dana called you," he says. "She wants you to call her back. Sexy voice, man."

At my lunch break, I slip into the spare office by the staff washroom and, with equal parts unease and anticipation, dial Dana's number. She answers after three rings.

"Mike. I need to see you. I'll pick you up at work and we'll go out for dinner in White Rock, at the Boathouse. Then we'll go for a long walk on the beach and watch the sunset."

I hesitate. The longer I'm sober, the harder it is to hang around still-drinking Dana. But I'm lonely. "Okay. Pick me up at the hospital back entrance on 94th Street at three o'clock. Right in front of Creekside."

At the end of the shift, I sit in the sun on the curb. I feel my back pocket for my cheque. Still there. I hear AC/DC pounding "Highway to Hell" as the little sports car pulls up with its top down.

"Well, hello, Mr. Pond. I see you're sitting outside one of our old haunts." Dana gestures to Creekside Withdrawal Management Centre.

I climb into the car and we cruise down King George Highway, straight into White Rock. Dana's eyes are glassy red; her breath smells of Smirnoff. I scan side roads where police might wait, ready to pounce on drunk drivers.

"Can you stop at the Scotiabank?" I ask. "I have to cash my cheque."

"Well, well, well." Dana grins. "Guess who's buying dinner tonight? It's about time you treated a pretty lady to a night out."

We pull up to the bank. I still have accounts with Scotiabank, where Rhonda and I hold a joint account for our lines of credit ... which are maxed out. My personal account sits empty. I make a mental note to make arrangements with my creditors. But not tonight. Tonight, after months of living on sixty dollars a month — all that remained from my welfare cheque after Rotten Randy deducted room and board — tonight, I celebrate.

I cash the entire amount. I count along as the smiling

teller stacks my bills: twenty fifties, ten twenties, one ten, a toonie, a loonie, two quarters, two dimes and two pennies. All there. I didn't need to cash the entire thing, but I did need to feel money again, to feel rich and substantial.

We walk into the Boathouse Restaurant, the first time I've been back since I stole the bottle of Glenfiddich last winter. As the hostess escorts us to our table, I drop my head and feel the hot flush of shame flash up the sides of my face. What if someone recognizes me? I should go up to the bar right now, admit my guilt and pay them back for the bottle of booze.

But do I have that kind of money right now? Shouldn't I save the bulk of my cash to begin repaying my monstrous debt? Morality and practicality tussle. I stay put, rooted at the table by embarrassment.

Our fish and chips arrive. I survey the food mounded on my plate, two giant portions of halibut lightly battered and fried to perfection, with fresh-cut fries, sea salt sticking to their glistening sides. Using my best Mission Possible manners, I shovel in bite after bite, plunging fry after fry deep into the ketchup. I slurp the salt off my fingers and mop up the grease running down my chin with my napkin. I wash it all down with gulps of cranberry juice and soda.

Dana orders one double Caesar after another.

I'm getting anxious.

"Let's go for a walk," I suggest.

"In a minute. I want another drink," Dana says.

"I think you've had enough, Dana. You're driving."

"Now that's funny, Mr. Two Back-to-Back Impaireds," Dana scoffs. "I think you're the last guy to be lecturing about drinking and driving." She polishes off yet another double Caesar.

As I watch her drink, I want one too. Badly now. But I'm also aware of a new sensation, a new feeling, almost a kind of yearning or longing for something else. Something normal.

Dana sucks back the last dregs of her drink and I wish I could wave a magic wand and be back with Rhonda and the boys. But that life's gone forever. I don't know that I'll ever stop missing it.

"Okay, Mr. Pond," Dana chirps. "I'm ready for our romantic walk along the beach."

I pull out my wad of money and pay the bill, $81.36. I count out four twenties and a ten and leave it on the table. It's positively painful to hand over that much money for one meal. Dana intertwines my arm in hers and I steady her out the door. We weave west along the teeming boardwalk toward the setting sun.

We wobble only a short distance toward the pier before Dana stops.

"Let's go to your house. I need to lie down for a while," Dana mutters.

Drunk, she slips behind the wheel. I look at her skeptically.

"That's my new car. No one drives it but me," she slurs.

My mind leaps back to that awful night almost a year ago when Dana pulled the knife on Sean, the night of my third impaired charge. The night the Mike-and-Dana train wreck began. When will it end?

Dana drops in behind the wheel and we make a quick and erratic dash back to the house. Dana collapses diagonally on the king-size bed, belly down, spread-eagled, one leg dangling over the edge. A pretty flip-flop slips off her pretty foot.

Passed out. Thank God.

I slump on the old couch in the living room. The gouged old hardwood floors have felt many hard boots, generations of sofas and coffee tables. I wait in the dark, quiet except for the snores soft and even in the bedroom, as random vehicles glide by on Russell Avenue and the neighbour's dog barks.

Why, with Dana asleep mere feet away, do I feel lonelier than ever?

Just past midnight, Dana comes to, groggy.

"I've got to go," she mumbles. "Thank you for dinner, Mr. Pond. Remember to meet me at Burrard Station next Sunday morning at eleven. We'll watch the Gay Pride Parade then go to the beach. Don't forget to bring your bathing suit. I'm going to wear the coral bikini I bought when we went to Whistler last summer. Bye bye."

I sit silently and watch as she waves and blows me a thoughtless kiss.

I have to break up with her. Which is a joke, because we're not even together. She's with Stu. Every time I ask about him, she's evasive. Watching her drink while not drinking myself gets more and more difficult. I'm torn between talking her into treatment and swiping her drink and polishing it off myself. We can't keep doing this to each other. In my shaky mental state, I'm not capable of truly being there for her, and while she's drinking, she's oblivious to anyone's needs but her own. I will go to the Gay Pride Parade, and that will be the end of it.

## 25

# THE LAST DATE

The week is uneventful. How I relish saying that. *The week is uneventful.*

With quiet and enormous satisfaction, I pay my rent, stock up on groceries, buy my first new clothes in a year, buy a bus pass and put the rest of the money in the bank. I begin to tackle my debt.

I introduce myself to the loans manager and ask her to tell me my credit rating. She scans her computer screen, looks me squarely in the eye and says one word. "Atrocious. Mr. Pond, if I were you, I'd file for bankruptcy."

The chorus recommending that course of action just keeps growing. But I can't. I won't.

I buy a cellphone at Best Buy, pay-as-you-go. I sail through another random urinalysis.

Dana phones every day to confirm our outing. It's as if she senses that the ground under this romantic relationship has shifted. I assure her I'll be there. And that, I remind myself, will be the end of it.

Friday, my last day of gradual return to work, I make my way back to the unit after a quick lunch in the hospital cafeteria up on the second floor. A small, frail man in a yellow hospital gown and blue paper slippers shuffles toward me. Something about him strikes me as oddly familiar. His one arm is in a sling, snug close to his chest; the other supports him on the wall as he painfully inches along. As I approach, the little man lifts his head and peers out of his left eye. The right one's swollen shut, a three-inch freshly sutured laceration across the brow. His head is bandaged, as if with a white toque, with one bloodied ear exposed. His nose shattered beyond recognition, he says in a nasal whisper, "Hey, Professor Pond. What are you doing here?"

The voice. I know the voice.

"Holy shit! Tom. What the hell happened?"

"Pretty nice, eh? I woke up in our bed last night to some son of a bitch smashing me with a framing hammer. They just released me. I'm going to kill that bastard."

The Tom "Guns" I knew a few months ago bears no resemblance to the one before me. He has lost at least forty pounds. His cheeks are hollow and grey, except for the blood and bruising.

"Rumour going around was that you were dead," I say. "I see that's not far from the truth. Come on, I'll buy you a coffee and something to eat."

As we walk to the cafeteria, Tom whispers, shamefaced, "I've been using now for a few months. We live in a crack house just off 96th. I owed this guy some serious money."

"Listen, Tom. I'm going to call Tim. He just started helping out at Mission Possible. You need to get clean and heal up."

Tim is a Fresh Start alumnus. A more resourceful and resilient guy is hard to find. Tim was a heroin addict and is now sober six years. When he was sixteen, he murdered his sister's abusive boyfriend — shot him in the heart with a bow and arrow. He was just a kid, but he did sixteen years' hard time at Stony Mountain Institution in Manitoba. When he got out, he lived homeless under a tarp in the forest in Abbotsford.

Tim got sober at Fresh Start, and to give back, he provides steadfast, unselfish service to anyone else in need. I call him now.

"Hi. Tim? It's Mike Pond. Tom 'Guns' is here at the hospital. He's been beaten almost to death. Would you be able to come and get him?" Tim says he's on his way and I hang up.

"Tom, sit tight. Tim will be here shortly. Stay at Mission Possible, and for God's sake, you gotta stay sober. You'll never survive another beating like that."

Friday draws to a close. Tuesday, after the long weekend, I become a full-time staff member. I did it. I'm on my way back.

The long weekend dawns sunny and gloriously hot. I wake up from my short and tortured sleep and head to Vancouver's West End, to the much-anticipated Gay Pride Parade. A transit officer works the platform, doing random checks for fare evaders.

I flash him my honestly gained transit pass and a wide smile. I grin ear to ear like an idiot. The transit officer, unaware I'm just so darn happy to be able to pay, grins back.

My Motorola pay-as-you-go reads 10:46 when I emerge from the train, head up the platform and spot Dana in a bright, frothy summer dress. She flashes me her stunner of a smile, and for a moment I'm mesmerized again. She deserves a life better than a drunk's.

We leave Burrard Station and walk the three blocks to Robson Street. There we thread our way through the throng, past a half-dozen young men clad only in shiny gold micro Speedos, spraying onlookers with Super Soakers. We bob and weave further through the screaming and laughing mob lined up along Robson in front of the shops. The mood is infectious. My morbid unease lifts.

The parade erupts in a display of exaggerated, over-the-top, in-your-face, fuck-you-if-you-hate-gays sexuality. I focus on Dana, for fear of losing her in the horde. She points to a small bistro with several outdoor patio tables with red umbrellas.

"Let's stop here and have a drink." She winks.

"No, let's stay and watch the parade."

A float blasting Madonna's "Like a Virgin" inches by. Young men decked out in white wedding gowns sing into wireless microphones.

Dana joins in the chorus, "Like a virgin. Touched for the very first time ..."

"Come on, party pooper." She pulls me into the bistro and sits at one of the tables. The waitress approaches.

"I'll have a Smirnoff lemon cooler and a double shot of vodka on the side." Dana rattles off her order without thinking. The waitress brings a bottled Smirnoff cooler and a tumbler half full of ice. Dana pours the foggy cooler into the glass, then splashes in the double shot of vodka. I've never noticed until now how ritualized drinking becomes for drunks. Each time, the same amount of ice, the precise measurement of liquid, the pause and the inevitable first sip — it all enhances the pleasure.

Dana downs half the glass in one gulp and then pays bright red lip service to my sobriety. "I hate to drink in front of you, Mr. Pond. You're doing so well."

I'm on the edge of not doing well at all. I'm ready to rip that cooler from her hands. But I don't.

As Dana gets drunk, the parade passes us by. We skip the beach.

We sit in silence on the long SkyTrain ride back to Dana's sister's place. We arrive there to find Doris on the back deck, trying to get some air.

"Hey," Dana says.

"Hi. Did you have a good time?" asks Doris.

"Yes, we did. I need a drink." Dana heads straight to the

kitchen. Bottles and glasses clink. Her bedroom door clicks shut.

I sit with Doris on the deck. She shakes her head and looks out into the backyard.

"She started drinking Friday," Doris sighs. "She just won't stop."

"She's an alcoholic, Doris. That's what we do."

Doris gets up stiffly. "I'm going to bed. I can't stand this anymore."

After waiting what seems an eternity for Dana to emerge, I knock on her bedroom door. No answer. I open the door. Dana lies face down, passed out in her coral bikini. A half-empty bottle of Smirnoff sits on the nightstand, an empty glass beside it.

I stand in the doorway for a long time before I walk over to the nightstand. My hands dangle by my thighs. My head turns slowly to Dana, unconscious on the bed, then back to the bottle.

I pick it up. I screw the lid on slowly. I want it now.

Four months sober, man. Don't do it.

Breathe, Mike. Just breathe.

The lid is on, tight.

I conceal the bottle behind some pots and pans in a kitchen cupboard. I close the cupboard and go sit in an easy chair. It's dark now.

From somewhere in the distance comes the unmistakable low rumble of thunder as a Harley Davidson creeps up the street. I peer out the front window and see an extremely large man dismount a stunning black and yellow chopper, shimmering in mirrored chrome.

Dana told me that Stu, the other man she's been seeing, was six foot eleven. She wasn't exaggerating. Stu is a mountain. He wears a black leather jacket, blue jeans and black Daytons — very large Daytons. He rests his black pan helmet on the extended handlebar of his chopper and strides toward the house. He has a mass of thick dark hair and hands the size of baseball mitts.

With some kind of death wish, I walk to the front door and swing it open. Stu freezes.

"Where's Dana," he booms.

I will myself not to shake.

I feign disinterest. "She's in bed passed out."

"Fuck! She's drunk." He looks me up and down, which doesn't take long. "You're that fucking Mike guy, aren't you? Is she seeing you again?" His eyes narrow.

Again? I wonder what lies she's been telling him.

"Looks like she's seeing us both."

"Fucking slut!" Stu stomps back to his spectacular Harley, kick-starts it, U-turns and yells through the engine's roar, "I'll be back." He accelerates up the hill.

I walk back into the kitchen and open the cupboard, retrieve the bottle from behind the pots and pans. I twist off the cap. And throw back one, then two big gulps. The sudden searing burn stuns my trembling gut. Within moments the familiar and oh-so-missed mellowness returns. How I hate myself.

I pour a few ounces of the Smirnoff into a tumbler and top it up with orange juice from the fridge. I sit back in the easy chair by the front window, ready for Stu's inevitable return. Within minutes, I hear the Harley thrump-brump back down the hill.

Stu climbs off his bike, grabs a stuffed green plastic garbage bag from the buddy seat and chucks it on the front lawn.

"Dana!" he bellows from outside. "Dana. Here's your all your shit. I want the fucking house keys. Now."

Dana's sister shuffles to the door in her pink velour

housecoat. "Dana!" she shrieks, and pounds on Dana's bedroom door. "Dana! Get up! Get up!"

Dana wakes up, peers out her bedroom window, runs into the front yard, still in her coral bikini. She glares at me as she passes. Busted.

"Stu." Dana fights to catch her breath. "What are you doing here?"

"You're a lying, cheating, drunken slut. Give me the house keys right now."

Dana flies into the house and returns with her purse, rummages through it and throws Stu the keys. He climbs onto his Harley and roars off again. Dana slinks back into the house.

"You son of a bitch. Look what you've done now," she hisses.

"Me. I'm just standing here."

"I hate you. I hate you." She swings at me with her fists and slams my face and chest.

Her sister walks away, disgusted.

Both fists clenched, Dana staggers back into her bedroom, banging and crashing around. "Where's my bottle? Where the fuck is my bottle?" Those blue eyes ablaze, she corners me in the kitchen. "What the fuck did you do with my bottle, you prick!"

She stomps back to the kitchen, spies the bottle on the counter, snatches it to her chest, then holds it out in front of herself and screams, "You've been drinking it! You son of a bitch! This is my bottle!" She supports herself on the wall with one arm as she returns to her room and whips the door shut.

It's seven minutes past midnight. I walk out of the house.

The night air is warm as I walk the streets for what seems like hours. Finally, I head to the Brentwood SkyTrain station. The city is quiet. I walk to the platform, drop down onto the long plastic bench by the tracks and wait. The trains are done running for the night. I look at my cellphone: 2:47.

I sit there on that plastic bench for almost six hours waiting for the first morning train. Six hours wide awake, wondering the whole time where I'd get my next drink. It's a holiday Monday. The train whirs into the station at 09:00. The car is empty, except for two teenage girls sitting together in the back seat texting, probably to each other.

Almost five months sober and I've blown it again. I need to drown my disappointment in myself. God, I need a drink.

# 26

# THE LAST BENDER

I step off the train at Surrey Central Station, walk straight to the beer and wine store, grab a four-pack of those Smirnoff coolers Dana drank at the bistro. These should last me the bus ride home. Then I pick up a twenty-sixer of Absolut, the really good stuff, as if anyone can tell the difference. I climb onto the 326 bus to White Rock, sit in the very back and twist the cap off the first cooler. By the time I arrive at the White Rock Central stop, all four coolers are gone. I slither off the bus with my precious Absolut clutched under my arm. I buy a two-litre carton of orange juice at the corner store and almost run to the little white house.

I wake up on the couch. I look around the house. The bottle of Absolut stands condemningly empty on the worn coffee table. A congealed puddle of orange something — is it vomit? — pools on the table and on the hardwood floor beside me. I snatch the bottle and drain the teaspoonful that's left into my mouth. I hack. I've got to go to the liquor store.

I bring home a forty-pounder of Grey Goose. I've got money. I'll buy the best.

I drink and black out and pass out and come to and drink more. Night becomes day becomes night after night after night of insanity and I know all the staffers on all the shifts at the twenty-four-hour liquor store. From deep in the recesses of my spongified brain, I drag out an image of a poster my boys wanted to put up around Penticton. My face captured like a mug shot under giant words: DO NOT LET THIS MAN BUY ALCOHOL. In their mounting anxiety, my teenaged sons concocted all manner of desperate measures to prevent me from drinking. It was Taylor's idea — he was working in a liquor store at the time. Now I wish they'd done it.

Will, a friend from AA, checks on me daily. He peers in the window as I lie on the couch. "You okay, Mike?" he says in his strong Polish accent. "You ready to stop today?"

"No, not today, Will," I say to the blurry-hazed shape in the window. He comes into the house with a bag of groceries.

"There's deli meat and bread here, Mike. Some first-class kolbassa sausage and Havarti cheese. You have to eat, Mike, or you will die. I have some Gatorade for you, too. You need the electrolytes. I'll leave it all in the fridge."

"Thanks a lot, Will. I'll have some later." I stare up at the ceiling.

The taste of food sickens me. The incessant drip-drip-drip of the tub faucet makes me want to rip out the plumbing with my bare hands.

The thousands of pilled threads on the cheap duvet dig into my skin. The damn sun is too bright. And no matter how much I scrub, the stench of vomit seeps from every pore.

My cellphone rings daily. It's work. I don't pick up.

How could I screw up work again? Will I end up in another recovery house?

Why can't I stay away from Dana? I have to see her. No — I have to never see her again.

I have to get up and walk to the liquor store.

One day, Big Jack and Don show up, two of the guys

living at Two-Finger Ted's, the White Rock sober house I should have moved into.

"Come on, Mike," says Don. "We're taking you to Fresh Start. It's August sixteenth. You've been drinking two weeks straight."

"No." I lay on the couch, one arm covering my eyes. "You're not taking me there. Let me be."

"Listen. We picked you up at the hospital the other night and brought you home." Big Jack steps into the living room. "A lady found you passed out in a lounge chair in her back-yard with a bottle of vodka still in your hand. You are really fucked up. You were talking about offing yourself. The cops took you to Peace Arch Hospital and they wanted to admit you to the psych ward, but you were too fucking drunk."

My cellphone rings. It's work. On the sixth ring, I pick up.

"Hello, Mike. It's Odette." She sounds annoyed, impatient. "We've been phoning you for almost two weeks."

"I've been very sick, Odette. Some kind of bug."

"HR received a letter today from Dr. Acres. A standard lab report from Peach Arch Hospital Emergency, positive for alcohol. You're suspended indefinitely without pay again. I don't like being lied to, Mike. The Review Committee will meet soon to decide what the next step is. You're probably looking at termination. I'm sorry, Mike."

It's starting to make sense now. If the cops took me from a woman's backyard to Peace Arch, of course they'd run lab work. I don't expect Fraser Health to give me a third chance. I suspect I'm done now.

I look up at Big Jack and Don from the couch.

"I'm going to the liquor store. Can you give me a ride, or at least pick me up a bottle?" I reach in my pocket, searching for money.

"You're really fucked up, Mike." Don shakes his head. "You're on your own, buddy."

I call my mother.

"The number you have dialled is blocked."

My mother blocked my calls. What have I been saying to frighten the old woman into silence this time?

My hands tremble out of control now as I drain the very last drop of vodka. Outside, I crouch down and — aha! — find a stray bottle holding a couple of ounces hidden under the deck. Still crouching, I swallow a sip.

As I carry my prize inside, I spy baby spiders crawling up the kitchen wall. As I move to swipe them away, they disappear.

*Clinical Notes — Mental Status Exam:*

*Patient appears unshaven and underweight, with dark circles under eyes. Psychomotor agitation. Extremities tremulous. Speech slurred and muffled. Mood depressed, fearful and anxious. Experiences visual and tactile hallucinations. Query Delirium Tremens. Suicidal ideation. Disoriented to time. Poor concentration. Insight fair. Judgment poor. Global Assessment of Functioning: 30/100 — major impairment.*

I retch, and the booze I just swallowed spews onto the floor.

I take another sip. Automatically rejected. Another trickle of vomit lands on the floor.

I try and try, and it just keeps coming back up. My system rejects every attempt, no matter how small the sip. What the hell?

I pour the last of the vodka down the sink. Must go to bed and sleep this off.

I come to on the couch. I roll over and grab my cellphone,

eyes straining to read the date: August 29, 2009, seven days since I took my last drink. This detox feels different. I've done it hundreds of times, and I know the drill. By now, the retching, writhing, chills and sweats should be history. I'd be wobbly and shaky for sure, but my energy should be coming back.

Not this time.

I can't take a deep breath without coughing. Sweat drips off my face. The pain in my head is so severe, it makes me vomit. Is this a migraine? Have I had a seizure?

I can't breathe. I have to get up and get to a doctor.

Sweat-soaked and cold, I sway and stop and prop myself up on the signpost at the corner of Russell Avenue and Johnston Street.

"You can do it, Mike, another thirteen steps," I propel myself forward. I keep stopping because one lung is on fire. Vehicles cruise up and down Johnson Street. As I rest I notice two brand-new pale green glass condo towers. Spectacular views of the bay, I bet. Maybe someday, in another life, I'll live there.

I left an hour ago and I'm only halfway there. I usually powerwalk this half-mile in ten minutes, max. I mark my painful progress with each power pole passed.

A spit-polished black BMW purrs by. The driver glances my way. A blend of sympathy and revulsion flashes across his face and he's gone. I drank vodka for twenty days straight. Next to no food. No sleep. I can only imagine how I look.

I gurgle with each inhale. Something has a stranglehold on my sternum. Something is seriously wrong.

Gasping for breath, I clutch the door frame at the entrance to Dr. Holic's clinic. His receptionist glances up, dashes around the desk to grab my arm and supports my dead weight as she hauls me into the examination room.

Dr. Holic rushes in. "Have you been drinking?" His face furrows with concern.

I can't answer because I can't breathe. Dr. Holic holds his stethoscope to my chest, then my back. He pauses on the lower left quadrant of my back. He taps my right side and produces a hollow resonant sound, like a drum. He taps the left side and we hear a thud. A dull, muffled thud.

"We need to get you to the hospital immediately." Dr. Holic tries to sound calm, but urgency and worry break through.

"Call the ambulance," he says to his receptionist. "Mr. Pond needs to go to Emergency."

The ambulance arrives in four minutes. We pull into the ER bay at Peace Arch Hospital, and the attendant rushes me through the automatic sliding doors.

The admitting nurse is waiting for me. "Temperature 40.4 degrees." She calls out my vitals to the ER doctor. "Pulse 110. Respirations 28 and shallow. BP 164 over 96."

The doctor presses his stethoscope to my back. "Your left lung is full," he says. "It's most likely empyema — complicated bacterial pneumonia. We will probably be transferring you to Surrey Memorial for surgery."

I aspirated vomit into my lung. While I holed up drinking for weeks, the infection advanced to a seriously dangerous stage. In their own version of a scared-straight program, the nurses are blunt. "Lots of guys who get this don't make it, Mr. Pond."

No. No. No. I'm not going out as a drunk, like my grandfather did, at fifty-six. This is not the legacy I wish for my sons.

And that is my last thought.

# 27

# DEATH'S DOOR

I wake up in a hushed room, bathed in a spaceship-like green glow. Machines whirl and gush and beep all around me. I glance and see tubes inserted everywhere.

I am in an intensive care unit. A nurse gazes down at me. Her mouth and nose are hidden behind a mask. She smiles and her eyes crinkle. I'm in isolation. Everyone who comes near adheres to strict infection protocol, partly to protect my immune-suppressed state, partly to protect everyone else.

I'm not dead. But I feel so bad, I'm not far from it.

Big Jack, Don and Tim crowd at the door. Robin and Owen don mask and gown. Tim shuffles nervously at the door. "You're gonna be okay, Mike," he says. "I just can't get any closer."

Tim is obsessive-compulsive and pathologically afraid of germs. Even setting foot in a hospital is a huge show of strength. Big Jack and Don hover anxiously above the bed.

"Mike, it doesn't get much worse than this," says Big Jack.

"Is this bottom enough yet?" Don laughs.

I fall once again into a deep, drug-induced sleep. I wake up to my own personal angel of mercy. Dana sits lotus-like at the bottom of the bed, a Smirnoff bottle clanking in her purse. She's semi-loaded but still manages to minister a sponge bath. She's unusually quiet.

"Just get better," she mumbles. "Please don't let it get any worse. It can't get any worse. You'll die."

After a ten-day stay at Peace Arch, the infection resists all treatment and I am transferred to Surrey Memorial, the hospital where I work. Or used to work.

My room is two floors directly above the adolescent psychiatric unit. Three chest tubes, inserted into my side and back, drain litres of blood-tinged fluid from my left lung. I go for X-rays and CT scans daily. On one of those daily gurney trips down to X-ray, as I lie in the hallway and wait my turn, Mark, the young APU nurse, walks by with a patient he's brought down for treatment. Our eyes meet. He can't quite get his head around what he sees. Neither can I. That life, that work, seems lost forever.

He approaches, obviously not actually sure it's me. I suspect I've lost at least thirty pounds since we last saw each other. I barely recognize myself either.

"Mike, is that you?"

"Hey, Mark, yeah, it's me."

His face floods with concern. He leans in close. "Get better, Mike," he says. "You're needed at work."

I'm needed at work. After all I've screwed up, Mark knows, intuitively, what I need to hear. And I think he actually means it.

The six-inch IV bag becomes the centre of my world. The promise of the silent, steady drip-drip-drip so far unfulfilled, I contemplate my death — not in a despairing suicidal manner, but with cool pragmatism.

How will I be buried? What's my final resting place, the small centuries-old cemetery in rural Ludlow, New Brunswick? Or should I have my ashes scattered across the mountains above Skaha Lake in the Okanagan? Who will pay for it? Rhonda, my ex, is so upset with me — *she* wouldn't.

At least I won't have to declare bankruptcy.

Dr. Ashton, my thoracic surgeon, holds out more hope than I do. Convinced it's just a matter of time until the potent antibiotics take hold, he delays surgery. "You're a tough guy, Mike, you just may pull through this without me having to open you up."

My mother is not convinced. She calls daily, likely thinking each will be our last conversation, crying and offering words of encouragement. How many calls to drunken sons can one woman make?

The AA guys never give up. Guys on their way to and from work, retired guys, guys still in rehab, all drop by, and I half-wonder whether I'm still alive because these guys resolutely refuse to let me go.

All but one. Angry Gord, who lent me the money for my original medical assessment with Dr. Acres, visits.

Don't need the money back, he had said back at Fresh Start. I'd been humbled by his offer. But you know what they say about offers that seem too good to be true.

Angry Gord scans me head to toe and checks the AccuVac container, almost full with red, mucus-like fluid.

"You look like shit," he says, and nods.

"Thanks, Gord. I feel like shit." I hack and spit.

"Do you have any money? I hear you were working again."

"I just used my last bit of cash." A sense of dread washes through me. "I asked Tim to buy me some minutes for my cellphone."

"But do you have any in your bank account?" Gord persists.

"I don't know. I haven't been able to check." I stare at the door and pray a nurse will walk in to check on me.

"That bitch hasn't been in to see you, has she?"

I cough steadily for over a minute. I can't get my breath.

Gord steps into the hallway and brings back a wheelchair. "Here, get in this. We're going for a walk."

"I don't know if I should, Gord. I have all this apparatus attached to me."

"Fuck that." He unwinds all the tubes, hooks the containers to the chair and wheels the IV pole over. "Here, hold this. I'm taking you down. Bring your wallet." We creep down the hospital corridor in silence to the elevator.

Gord stops the wheelchair in front of an ATM. He moves off to the side and watches over his shoulder, arms crossed.

I insert my bankcard and enter my PIN. Push the display balance option. $77.73. I withdraw sixty.

Gord comes over and I hand him the three twenties. He wheels me back to my room and disappears as I collapse yet again into a massive coughing fit.

"Mr. Pond, you look like you're at death's door. You look seventy years old."

It's Dana, drunk. Once again she curls like a cat at the bottom of my bed. She digs deep in her purse, pulls out a twenty-sixer of vodka and mixes it with a Red Bull.

"Do you mind if I have drink?" she asks and slurps her concoction.

"No, Dana, you go ahead." I watch her with an odd blend of sadness and resignation. I want to get better. I want her to get better. I know that will never happen as long as we are together.

I brace myself for the inevitable craving, the longing for just one sip that begins the downward spiral all over again, one that deepens the chasm between me and all that gives my life meaning and grace and sustenance. I can't play hockey anymore, because the team quit me. My niece doesn't talk to me anymore because I got too drunk to MC her wedding. I destroyed too many Christmases at my in-laws, Armond and Doreen's, bless their big hearts and ever-patient souls.

And always present, the image of Taylor, physically ejecting me out of my own home, his brothers and mum standing resolute behind him.

Wait for it — the urge to wrest that Red Bull from Dana's hand and gulp it down.

Wait. Nothing yet, but wait. Maybe it's just late because I've been ill.

I wait and watch and wait. And holy shit — I don't want a drink. I mean, I really don't want a drink.

Is this what Eli at Fresh Start means about finally surrendering? Is this the miracle my ex-in-laws and so many other others have been praying for? Or is this my mind and body simply saying we're done? Has my brain chemistry for some unknown reason suddenly become like normal people's?

Rhonda closing the door to Jonny's room after she kicked me out of the house, me coming to amidst the broken glass of the windshield of my crushed brand-new Honda Ridgeline truck, the battering ram I used to break into Dana's friend's house, swiping the booze from the Boathouse, being finger-printed, Belinda taking me back to Mission Possible, the putrid whiff of Psycho Jordan's festering leg, crouching down in ditches to gather empties for bus fare — moment after moment from my years of drunken insanity fly past me now, fast-forwarding through five years of carnage.

I've known what it is to resist the cravings. I've known what it is to fold like a cheap tent and down a twenty-sixer as soon as it stands naked in front of me. But I've never experienced this before, no craving at all. Period.

Euphoria, elation, relief and maybe finally peace — feelings totally foreign tumble over me one after another, slam me into the boards, knock the wind out of me.

I struggle to compose myself as Dr. Holic strides in the room. He looks pointedly at Dana and says, "I hope your intentions are good. This is a good man."

I feel tears well up in my eyes. Somewhere in me, I have to believe, there is a good man.

Dana slides off the bed, pecks me on the cheek and mutters that she's got to get to work.

In the hospital, life takes on its own tenuous rhythm to the soundtrack of the suction machine. IV antibiotics change on schedule. Doctors and interns huddle over CT scans and X-rays, perplexed as to why the infection seems so intractable. Each day they discuss whether to operate, which carries its own risks, or whether to wait for my body to fight back. The longer surgery is delayed, the greater the potential for long-term lung damage.

Three weeks into intensive care, I sense a barely perceptible shift. I feel slightly more able to breathe. I return from my daily CT scan to find Dr. Ashton and his phalanx of interns.

"Looks like you've turned the corner, Mike," he smiles. "This bug is finally backing off."

By the time I'm released, over five litres of blood-tinged fluid have drained from my left lung.

As I sign my release forms, I shake the thoracic surgeon's hand. "Thank you, Dr. Ashton. You did a great job. You saved my life."

"You're welcome, Mr. Pond. A lot of people don't make it from this. You are a very fortunate man. I pray you have had your last drink of alcohol."

"Thanks. So do I."

"Here's a prescription for you." He hands me the paper. "A final regime of oral antibiotics and Tylenol 3 for pain."

"Thanks, doctor." I stuff it in my pocket. "I won't take the T3s. They're restricted."

Max gave up the little white house while I was in hospital. His girlfriend dumped him. Big Jack, from AA, told me he relapsed the day before his fourth sobriety birthday. I have

$17.73 to my name. The hospital social worker cannot find me a home in a shelter. I ask Don from AA to do the unthinkable: ask Rotten Randy to take me back at Mission Possible. I used to think I'd rather die than go back there. I never thought I'd actually have the opportunity to make that choice.

I choose Mission Possible. I choose life.

# 28

# FIFTY-SIX

September 26, 2009. An AA guy drives me back to Mission Possible. I walk in and Rob, my unwavering supporter, my sidekick in bottle scavenging, my fellow tortured New Brunswicker, greets me and shakes my hand. His grip is firm like he doesn't want to let go. "It's good to see you're okay, old man." His voice breaks.

Several guys sit out back smoking. Must be new clients, as I don't know any of them.

As I shuffle past the little office by the front door, Ken looks out and laughs. "Escaped the Grim Reaper again, eh, Pond? You're a lucky bastard."

Rotten Randy sits at the desk in front of Ken, grins without looking up and begins to rail. "I told you. I told you you'd fuck up. You owe me a month's back rent, Pond. Ken will take you to Welfare tomorrow. You still have an open file. Just get a note from your doctor."

"I have a letter here from the lung specialist at the hospital. He says I'm unable to work indefinitely until I have medical clearance. I'll take it with me."

And then, as per house protocol, I hand over my prescriptions. Every day, the pharmacist delivers the precise amount of meds needed for each man. Sure is an expensive way to administer meds, as there will be the inevitable dispensing fee for each pill, but it kind of makes sense given that we are all addicts of some kind. Don't want too many drugs lying around the house.

Randy dismisses me with a backhand wave.

"Here's some mail for you." Ken tosses an envelope at me. "Looks like a letter from your work. Or what used to be your work. Ha ha."

Fraser Health Authority, reads the envelope. I don't even want to open it.

"They've called a few times," Ken says. "We just said you were still in the hospital."

I trudge down the stairs to the claustrophobic, dingy, stinky dorm. In the corner on a lower bunk, a rotund guy lies on his back with an open paperback perched on his face.

"Hello, Pond. Eli's right, eh? Get a job, get a girl, get drunk."

Dangerous Doug. I last saw him when he showed up on my ward at work a drunken, blubbering idiot, begging for my forgiveness for telling Dana I'd committed suicide.

"Doug. What are you doing here?"

"Sick. Detoxin'. I hate this fucking place already. Buncha rejects from Fresh Start."

Sleep is fitful this first night back as I follow the bouncing ball of my fucked-up life around my brain. I'll be fired. I'll lose my licence to practise. Go to court and prison. My financial disaster. My divorce. My alienated sons. My estranged friends. But I'm buoyed by my secret: all of this shit is going on, but I don't want a drink.

In the morning, Ken takes me to the welfare office. I get a cheque to pay the rent for October. My new social worker hands me another cheque, held from August. I can pay off Randy and have an extra $120. I should feel relief. I should feel thankful. But I don't.

I sit on my bunk alone in the dorm. With trepidation, I finally open the letter from the Fraser Health Authority.

*Mr. Michael Pond,*

*The Review Committee has decided that you must complete another independent medical assessment to assist in making a determination with respect to your employment status, as well as your competence to practise as a Registered Psychiatric Nurse and a Registered Social Worker. Please contact Dr. Richard Flannigan at 604-528-1881 as soon as possible to schedule this assessment. Upon receipt of Dr. Flannigan's assessment report, the Review Committee will meet with you to make its determination. The costs of this assessment will be covered by your employer — Fraser Health Authority. Please contact me with the appointment date.*

*Sincerely,*

*Colleen Slater, BScN, RN*

*Occupational Health Nurse*

*Fraser Health Authority*

I hold my breath. The letter slides to the floor. Unbelievable. I get a third chance.

I dash to the client phone in the closet and dial the number.

"Dr. Flannigan's office," the receptionist says. "How can I help you?"

"Hello. My name's Michael Pond. My employer has requested I contact you to schedule an assessment with Dr. Flannigan."

"Yes." I hear a keyboard clicking as the receptionist types.

"Mr. Pond. We received the referral from Fraser Health Authority. Dr. Flannigan has been waiting for your call."

"I'm sorry, I've been in the hospital. I can come in any time. As soon as possible, please."

October ninth is the first available date. I lunge for it.

"I'll be there. Thank you, so much."

Rob yells, "Hey, Pond! Come up here quick. Randy says you owe him more money."

Fuck. I set the phone down and jump up the stairs two at a time. By the time I hit the top, my chest constricts and the endless succession of coughs begins, almost drowning out the first bars of "Happy birthday to you. Happy birthday to you. Happy birthday, Crazy Mi-ike. Happy birthday to you."

A chorus of guys crowd around the dining-room table, singing to a large rectangular chocolate cake with a 50 made of white sprinkles circled by six little pink and white birthday candles.

"We couldn't afford that many candles," laughs Rob. "You're too fucking old, Pond."

"Rob baked you the cake, Mike," says Wayne. "It's from scratch. He scrounged everything. My wife donated the icing, sprinkles and candles from home. Stuff left over from my daughters' birthday parties. Happy birthday, old man."

I blink back tears as I scan the circle of men. Men who've become my only friends, men who went to such extraordinary measures to mark a day I'd prefer to forget. For a flicker, I see them all dressed like a horde of eight-year-old buccaneers, brigands and a few maidens.

Brennan's eighth birthday party, featuring three Captain Hooks. The patio table's transformed into a cardboard schooner. Cooper, our miniature schnauzer, wears an eye patch. He eats the end of a hotdog hanging from the hand of Blackbeard. A Jolly Roger flaps atop the patio umbrella pole. A couple of old Captain Morgan rum bottles filled with root

239

beer sit on the table. Plastic mugs clutched two-handed in midget pirate hands. I laugh as I raise a toast with my rum and Coke — to Rhonda, the best damn pirate birthday party planner in town.

As is ceremony, I make a wish and make a show of blowing out the six pink and white candles. I wish for my old life back.

# 29

# THE UNIVERSE CUTS
# ME A BREAK

I go to my appointment with Dr. Flannigan, the addictions specialist the Fraser Health Authority requires me to see.

He's a pleasant Irishman in his early fifties, in Canada twenty-three years but he sounds like he's just off the boat. His accent charms and disarms. He's been interviewing me for over an hour and it's still going strong.

"You have quite an incredible story, Mr. Pond. We must take a break. Complete these tests. I will check your provincial pharmacy record, and we will finish up the assessment at eleven thirty."

After forty-five minutes, Dr. Flannigan returns with a report in his hand.

"We have a problem, Mr. Pond." The lilt is diminished.

"What is it, Dr. Flannigan?"

"You've been taking narcotics."

"No." I shake my head. "I haven't taken anything. Just my prescribed meds: Celexa, trazodone."

"Yes, I see that here. But you also filled a prescription for thirty Tylenol 3s on September twenty-eighth."

"No, I didn't."

"Well, it says right here you did." He taps the report in his hand.

"No, I didn't." I'm adamant, trying to keep a lid on my mounting frustration. And then it dawns on me. That fucking Randy. He's notorious for helping himself to meds prescribed for other clients at Mission Possible. *He* filled my prescription.

"Dr. Flannigan, clearly it has been filled, but not by me. I promise you. The guys who run the recovery house I'm in fill all the prescriptions. The medications get delivered to the house every day."

"Mr. Pond, I've worked with addicts for over thirty years. I find it very hard to believe your story. I will have to indicate in your report that you have been taking narcotics."

"NO! Dr. Flannigan. I'm telling you the truth. I have not taken *one* of those pills."

He looks me hard in the eye. A sad, wizened expression softens his face. "I'm sorry, Mr. Pond. I will send the report to your employer by the end of next week. It is up to them to give you a copy if you so desire. Goodbye."

"Can I ask please that you consult with Dr. Acres? He's been working with me for months now."

"Yes. I was planning on doing that anyway."

"Thank you." I trudge out of the office. Shock and fury and a surge of self-pity engulf me as I stand in the rain and call Grant, an AA guy, to pick me up. Why can't the universe cut me a break? Here I am toeing the line, trying to do the next right thing, as my son Brennan exhorts, not cheating, not drinking, and life still doesn't get better or easier.

I fill Grant in as we head back to Langley. He listens, dumbfounded.

"Those bastards filled my prescription for T3s. That pharmacist in Abbotsford delivers my four pills daily as prescribed. They charge a dispensing fee each time." My brain, firing on all cylinders now, puts the pieces together. "Of course the pharmacist must be in cahoots with Randy and Ken. Randy takes a cut. That's quite the racket. And Ken gets all the narcotics he wants. No wonder he sleeps all fucking day."

I don't say a word to anyone when I get back to the house. I know all I will get is denial. I march straight to the phone to call Dr. Acres. He must know about the Tylenol 3 prescription being illegally filled and sold.

On Monday I call Bob Fallows, my new lawyer, and fill him in. When I first called Fallows, he shut me down. "I don't do legal aid," he says. "It's just not worth it. I end up making at best fifty bucks an hour, and it's labour intensive."

I told him my story. He listened without a word, and finally said, "I'm a recovered alcoholic, now twenty-two years sober. I'll take your case. Stay sober, stay in rehab and I'll meet you in the lobby of the Surrey courthouse in a few months."

"Mike, we have a court date now," he says. "December second. You must plead guilty. You have no defence."

"I know. I want to plead guilty." I want to plead guilty because I *am* guilty. Guilty as hell.

"Okay. I want you to give me a detailed written list of all the treatment you have received right from day one. And write me a biography of your battle with alcoholism. Just stay sober. And stay in that place you're in. Get a good report from the guy who runs the place. I know he's an asshole, but stay on his good side. And we'll get a good report from Dr. Acres. He's got a lot of clout. With the right judge, you might be looking at just three to six months."

"Just!"

"Or less. You never know what's going to happen. The Criminal Code says minimum thirty days, and with the accumulation of alcohol-related charges and driving while suspended, it doesn't look good."

Wednesday, October fourteenth, I sit in Dr. Acres' waiting room, still brimming with anger and frustration over the damning pharmacy record. In he walks.

"Good morning. Sobriety date?" Every meeting begins this exact same way. He's smiling. That can't be right. He must have talked to Dr. Flannigan by now.

"August twenty-third."

"Excellent. I talked with Dr. Flannigan this morning. You remember when you came in last week and we took a urine sample."

Yes. Oh-my-gawd-yes, I see where this is heading.

"It came back negative," says Dr. Acres. "Exactly the time you were supposedly taking four T3s a day. Impossible. I've informed Dr. Flannigan. That will be reflected in his report. Clearly, someone else filled that prescription. You see, there is a God, Michael. As well, Dr. Flannigan and I will be reporting this activity to the College of Pharmacists."

"Oh my God!" I smile, a huge grateful grin. "Thank you, Dr. Acres."

"I also received a letter from your lawyer. I will write him a favourable report. Just keep doing what you're doing. Stay clean and sober. Come see me every two weeks. Go to at least three meetings a week. Talk to your sponsor. See you in two weeks."

Vindication changes everything. I embrace sobriety. I religiously attend AA meetings in White Rock, sometimes two or three a day. I ask Robin, a reformed heroin addict, to be my sponsor.

For the next few months, I'm bolstered by his unwavering support. Knowing how much I despise Mission Possible, Robin regularly rescues me. Breakfasts, lunch, dinner, coffees, phone calls at all hours of the day or night, Robin is there. His quiet belief in God and his steadfast commitment to the AA program ground me. He listens without judgment.

"Just stick with the program, Mike," he reminds me, often. "Believe that it's in God's hands." Part of me believes it's in God's hands. But the seasoned practitioner lying dormant in me knows it's ultimately up to me. Yes, I need the social supports, but my own cognitive distortions sabotage any sense of hope or optimism. "I will never be successful again," "I will never have a loving mate," "I am too damaged." The first step in cognitive behavioural therapy is to become aware of self-defeating thoughts and negative beliefs about one's self. I determine that I will become my own therapist. I will work with and for Mike Pond. I construct my own treatment plan:

1. *Identify the problems: (a) depression, (b) anxiety.*
2. *Establish the goals: (a) reduce severity of symptoms, (b) improve self-regulation of mood.*
3. *Treatment approach: (a) cognitive behavioural therapy, (b) medication as prescribed, (c) social support.*

That social support is AA. The invisible web of AA support weaves around me, preparing me for the worst still to come — prison. Steve, an ex-cop, Grant, an gnarly loyal old Irishman, and Tim comprise my personal holy trinity. I stay at Grant's house often, just to be away from Mission Possible, to get a glimpse of what a real life could look like one day.

I force myself to go for walks. I catch my negative self-talk and self-defeating thoughts. I restructure them into positive, optimistic thoughts — cognitive restructuring.

November arrives, and the grey, dark, rainy days bleed into one another. This weather usually sends me into a funk, but not this time. This month, I'll appear before the review committee at Fraser Health. This time, I believe they will support me.

Next month, in December, I'll go to court and inevitably to jail. I've accepted my fate. I accept that it's all out of my hands. I will get through this, and I will learn from it.

*When are you going to surrender your will? Have your surrendered yet, guy? You won't get sober under you've surrendered.* I now know the meaning of Eli's and Josh's endless hectoring.

Life at Mission Possible seems strangely more tolerable too, because Rotten Randy has not been seen for days. One day, a group of us sit at the table playing cards. Young John, who was here a year ago and just came back, shares the news. "Did you hear? Randy is at Fresh Start. He relapsed," he says. "One day he's on the cover of the *Province*, saviour of the down and out. Next day he's one himself, living in a recovery house."

I should be happy that Rotten Randy has fallen off the wagon. But that kind of thinking is mean-spirited, and I'm growing to believe what goes around comes around. Neil rarely comes to the house anymore. Ken sleeps constantly, emerging from his room only to eat.

Tim takes over Mission Possible. He and his partner lobby for donations and sponsorship. Almost immediately the food improves. The night he takes over, we eat roast beef, gravy, mashed potatoes and broccoli.

Angry Gord facilitates our group meetings. I've seen him in AA meetings over the past few months, but we haven't spoken to each other. This is our first close encounter since he wrote me off for dead in the hospital and came to collect on his debt.

At the group meetings, Gord practises his own brand of confrontational therapy. "How do you feel about driving drunk, Mike? Do you feel guilty about the fact that you could have killed someone? Do you sleep at night, Mike? Do you have any shame or remorse at all?"

"Gord, drop this. Of all the things I've done drunk, driving is the one for which I feel the most shame. Drop it."

Gord is nowhere near done. He reaches into his briefcase and pulls out a multiple-page document. I immediately recognize it — Dr. Acres' initial assessment report. Gord asked me for a copy of it. Since he'd paid for it to be done, I thought it only fair that he get a copy. I didn't think much of it then. I sure as hell do now.

"Put that away, Gord! It's totally inappropriate. It's private — between me and my doctor."

Gord ignores my protests and reads out loud. "Mr. Pond was self-referred at the recommendation of his professional governing body for an assessment of his competency to practice —"

I lunge at him and snatch the report out of his hands.

"Don't you fucking ever try something like this again!" I tear the report to pieces and stomp out of the meeting. I still owe Gord over a thousand dollars. I vow to pay him back — every penny. I shake with anger. In a proper treatment centre, no one would dream of treating a client like this.

Monday, November twenty-third: I sit with the Review Committee, to see whether I get my job back at Surrey Memorial. This time I wait not with dread, like before, but with anticipation. For once I've done everything right.

The same members are all here around the table.

"Michael," begins the HR rep. "We know that you have been clean and sober three months. You have been following the agreement conditions since your unfortunate relapse in the summer. Dr. Flannigan's report is favourable. The committee has agreed that you may commence another gradual return-to-work program in two weeks, December seventh. How does that sound?"

I fight back the tears and compose myself before whispering, "Thank you. Thank you."

Just one obstacle — by December 7, I'll likely be in prison.

"I would like to delay my return till the New Year. I have some personal matters that I'll need to deal with over the next month or more."

My manager, Kay, checks her calendar. "Okay, how does Monday, January third, look? If that's not enough time, let us know and we can postpone."

Oh dear God, please let that be enough time. That would mean only a month in prison. That would mean getting off lightly.

# 30

# YOUR HONOUR

It's 9:33 in the morning and I'm sitting on the narrow, finely polished bench outside the courtroom and wait for Bob Fallows, my lawyer. I am about to begin what is without a doubt the worst day of my life. Barring a miracle — and I've been running pretty short on those — I'm going to prison. All night, I rehearsed what I'll say to the judge.

*Your Honour, I am guilty of everything as charged. I just thank God I didn't hurt or kill anyone.*

*Your Honour, thank God, I never hurt or killed anyone. In my current sober state, driving drunk is indefensible.*

*Your Honour; Your Honour; Your Honour.*

Anxious questions interrupt my rehearsals. What will my boys say when their friends ask them where I'm spending Christmas? How will my mother get through it? How will I get through it? I began my career working in institutions. I know what goes on in there.

My guts churn. We are scheduled to appear in twenty-seven minutes. Bob Fallows weaves his way through the waiting crowds in the lobby of the Surrey courthouse. Bob is about my size, and I suspect we're close to the same age. He cuts a rumpled Columbo-like figure as he shuffles my way.

I wear an oversized, decades-old hand-me-down suit, shiny with wear. I snagged it and a pair of dress shoes after an elderly widow dropped off her dead husband's clothes at Mission Possible. She told us he was a big man. The suit's sleeves hang past my knuckles. I shuffle along in bankers' shoes that are three sizes too big. My precious Rockports, the last vestige of the man I used to be, were stolen off me at Fresh Start.

My Rockports — I remember when I'd poured myself off the Greyhound into the Downtown Eastside and rummaged through my duffle bag to find something warm and water-proof to wear. What had I packed? Padded biking shorts; a basketball pump; one running shoe and a single bike shoe, both for the left foot. Clearly, a drunk had packed my bag. Then, finally, the beautiful pair of shiny black waterproof Rockports. They say you can tell a lot about a man from his shoes. Wonder what mine say about me now?

Everywhere around me, lawyers mill about, engaged in urgent conversation with their clients, voices muted, bodies taut. The high ceiling underscores the sense of import. I see young Max, my former roommate at the little house in White Rock. We glance ruefully at each other. I heard from the other guys he's facing another impaired driving charge. After his fiancée broke up with him, he launched on an anguished post-break-up tear and crashed his truck, four years of sobriety evaporated. I wonder what it would feel like to be sober that long. I can't even imagine it.

"I just gave the judge a copy of the biography you sent me," Bob says as he sits down on the bench beside me. "I've had guys write these bios for twenty-five years. I hope to God the judge is as impressed with it as I was. But I don't hold out much hope. BC's got zero tolerance for drunk driving now. You are going to prison."

I slump back against the hard polished wood. Over my years as a therapist, I often asked clients what they had to look forward to. It's a way of gauging psychological hardiness. It is in the absence of hope that people suffer the worst despair. I ask myself now. I can't think of anything. I am empty. I only exist in this moment of dread.

We file in through the double doors. The courtroom is packed; an assembly line of petty crime waits to be processed. There's a steady murmur of low conversation and the constant coming and going of red-suited prisoners as they are processed from remand.

My turn.

I stand alongside Bob Fallows before the judge. I peer up at him. He scrutinizes me over the rims of his glasses, then leafs through a slew of papers before him. I notice the lined notepaper of my handwritten bio. He glances at me, then the documents, then back at me. Our eyes meet, and in his, I see compassion.

"Mr. Pond," he starts. "You have a very tragic and compelling story, and it is a miracle you are still alive; however, the law says that it is mandatory that I send you to jail. Do you have anything to say before I pass sentence?"

"Thank you, Your Honour." Here we go. "I take full responsibility for my actions. I thank God every day that no one was hurt or killed."

"Mr. Pond, when I review your driving record, I am taken aback. Until 2007, you have no previous infractions other than the odd speeding ticket. However, in the last two years you have amassed a terrible record. Twelve offences: all related to alcohol — *three* impaired convictions alone in an eight-month period."

Sweat beads on my brow. I can't tell if the courtroom is overheated or I am. I take a quick look over my left shoulder. Is everyone hearing this? Or are they all so fixated on their own fates, they've got no interest in mine. Please God, let that be the case.

The judge continues. "Mr. Pond, you have a very, very

serious problem. I hope you maintain your sobriety. In any event, I am sentencing you to thirty days in jail and a two-year suspension of your driver's licence. I suspect that the Superintendent of Motor Vehicles will take it away even longer. That decision is out of my hands. Good luck, Mr. Pond."

And that's it. He turns his attention to the next of dozens of cases he'll pass judgment on today.

My shoulders drop and my arms weigh heavy at my sides. A warm, tingling sensation floods the back of my neck, and I notice my breath for the first time this morning. Shallow and rapid — I'm ready for flight. But I've got nowhere to go. I fight the urge to bolt out of the courtroom. With a jerk of her head, the sheriff standing adjacent to the prisoners' docket beckons me over. Cool sweat spills over my tight shirt collar.

"Inmate for processing," she barks by rote.

*Dead man walking* is what I hear. My life collapses into itself.

As if in a trance, I proceed down a concrete staircase to a dimly lit, cavernous tunnel. I sense we're underground. Covered security cameras stand like sentinels. I remember observing prisoners from the other end of those cameras when I worked for Federal Corrections in the eighties. Now I am one of the rats in the maze.

Straight ahead, a large Plexiglas enclosure holds several officers in blue uniforms in front of computer monitors that sit on a sixteen-foot-long half-circle desk. One gestures to one of three cells along the off-white concrete wall to the right. "In there."

I am in jail.

# 31

# THE FRASER
# REGIONAL
# CORRECTIONAL
# CENTRE

I survey my cellmates: a motley crew of prisoners dressed in drab-red cotton pants with elastic waistbands and matching T-shirts. No belts here. Belts are weapons and make very effective nooses. Who here has potential to hurt me?

"Pond, come with me," orders an officer with two stripes on each of his powder blue sleeves. I estimate that he is in his mid-fifties; he has grey receding hair — close to retirement. Do I detect a nugget of empathy for a fellow old warhorse?

"You don't belong here, Pond," he says as we walk. "Thank the fuck it's only thirty days. Do your own time. Don't piss anyone off, and you'll get outta here in twenty without getting shit-kicked or ass-fucked. Some of the perverts like old fuckers like you."

*Do your own time.* I first heard that expression from kids I counselled in juvenile detention, jail-slang for "mind your own business." Take care of your side of the street and don't interfere with or bother anyone else. Keep your nose clean and it won't get busted.

The guard escorts me to another wing, with a cordoned-off area. A twelve-foot-by-four green laminated counter separates two officers from the rest of the population.

"Strip naked, lay all your clothes here and shower from head to toe." Drumming his palm on the counter, a young officer about Brennan's age begins to process me.

I am mute. In shock, I dump the ancient suit on the counter with the rest of my belongings and submit to the humiliation of a public shower. I know worse is to come.

After I pat dry with an institutional white towel, the close-to-retirement officer appears again, this time sporting powder blue vinyl gloves. With practised precision, he inspects me head to toe. First front. Then back.

"Bend over. Spread your cheeks, and not the ones on your face. We want to see if you're hooping any contraband."

Hooping is the preferred way of bringing drugs into jail. And any old hoop will do. Guys like me are prime hooping candidates for the heavies to mule drugs and money into the joint. We're low risk of being busted. And besides, they can rent a hoop real cheap when accompanied by the encouragement of a framing hammer applied full force to the kneecap. For a man whose life has been law-abiding, this indignity is indescribable.

Freshly showered, inspected and newly attired in my red BC Corrections garb, I follow the officer back to the holding cell. It is full now with several men recently transferred in from other facilities.

In waddles Tom "Guns," accompanied by two rather large gentlemen, all dressed in red. Like a periscope, Tom's head swivels on his thick neck — past me, then a sharp jerk back. "Holy shit! Mike Pond. What are you doing here?"

Tom keeps popping up in my life, first as a troubled

fifteen-year-old client in youth detention in 1991. Then last year, when he introduced me to the couch of willingness in the Fresh Start recovery house. And finally, just a few months earlier, when I'd returned to work at Surrey Memorial, where he was hobbling down the hall toward me: tiny, frail and strung out on crack, beaten to a pulp in a drug deal gone bad.

Now he's back in prime fighting form. Tom stands five foot two, made up of two hundred pounds of solid muscle. He is built like an oak tree trunk, and I know for a fact he can one-punch anyone into unconsciousness. But Tom shows no mercy; he rarely stops after one. Like so many addicts, he has an uncanny capacity to survive.

Once again, with that same engaging smile, thirty-four-year-old Tom asks, "How much time did you get, Mike?"

"Thirty days."

"No way! For sure I thought you'd've gotten at least six months. The judge musta liked you. Just do your own time, dude. I know a lot of guys in FRCC. Just tell 'em you're a friend of Tom 'Guns.' Before you know it, you'll be out. Sucks we'll be in here for Christmas, though, eh?"

A guard comes to the cell and calls out, "Pond. You're going upstairs."

"See you again, Tom. Good luck, eh?" I pat him on the shoulder.

"Luck's got nothin' to do with it, Mike," says Tom. "You're a really smart guy. Just keep an eye out for the fuck-heads — you know who they are."

I force a smile and flash him a peace sign as the guard leads me to an elevator around the corner. Tom smiles back, shakes his head and gives me the finger.

"Here. You're going up. You'll stay the night, then straight to FRCC in the morning."

Cradling my only belongings — a towel, toothbrush and

soap — I step into an elevator with several other guys. All in drab red. No guards in elevators. I discover later that some guys step out of jail elevators with broken noses or curled up in the fetal position with smashed testicles. The doors open and we all file into an open range with cellblocks circling a central guard desk. A muscular young blue-shirt assigns us to our cells. A blue shirt signifies a lower-ranking officer, white shirt — senior officer.

A large round schoolhouse clock behind the blue-shirt reads 5:02. A stainless steel, six-foot-high institutional hot food cart on little wheels arrives, and all the men clamour toward it. Two inmates hand out the trays. I remain sitting in one of the plastic chairs. I don't want to eat. A skinny guy in his mid-forties with dirty blond, close-cropped hair approaches me with two trays in hand.

"Hey, man." He motions for me to take a tray. "You, me and couple other guys are heading to Fraser Regional Correctional Centre in the morning. Have something to eat. It tastes like shit, but you gotta eat. Get used to it or you'll starve."

"No thanks." I shake my head. "No appetite."

"You'll get used to the food. No better at FRCC. I've been there, twice. My name's Lee."

"Mike."

"What's your story?"

"Drunk driving."

"They put you in jail for that!"

"It's a little more than just that."

Lee informs me that he has spent half of his life in jail. In and out since he was fourteen. All non-violent crimes, B & E's, theft, trafficking — all drug-related. He's easygoing and friendly. For the first time today I relax a bit. Lee is about six foot two with the build of a swimmer but the dental work of a crackhead. His mouth smells as bad as it looks.

"There are some real sick sons a' bitches in these joints,

Mike." He doesn't need to speak the name. The notorious serial killer Willy Pickton is upstairs in the top floor, an entire unit to himself. Everyone wants him dead.

"You and me," Lee says, "we'll get a cell together at FRCC. I know most of the guards. We'll both go to open custody. A lot more freedom. Open cells most of the time. Not as many goofs and GTs." That's prison speak for gangster thug.

"I'm pretty wasted, Lee. I'm going to my cell." I stand up to leave.

"In here, call it your 'house,' Mike. You won't sound like such a fresh fish. A greener." Lee grins.

The houses haven't changed since I worked with adult inmates twenty-five years ago. Battleship grey, semi-gloss, oil-based paint on the walls, ceiling and floor, including the steel bunk beds, with the all-too-familiar two-and-a-half-inch-thick black vinyl workout mats for mattresses. The sheets never fit, bundling into a wrinkled roll somewhere between your hips and armpits. No matter how tightly I cinch them under the mattress, I wake with my face plastered to the sticky vinyl.

*You don't belong here, Pond.* I echo the guard's words to myself. But a part of me knows I do.

Chin propped on the heel of my hand, my fingers anxiously toggle my cheek. My elbow goes numb as I peer out the narrow barred window. It's open to the max, three and a half inches. Outside it's dark, raining hard. A variety of vehicles volley in and out of a spot lit parking lot.

I lie on the bed and unbidden memories pounce. Taylor wakeboarding on the calm water. Four-year-old Jonny perfecting his slapshot. Brennan and I flying down Big White on freshly waxed snowboards. The chocolate-sweet smell of Rhonda's ranger cookies baking in the kitchen. The searing sand at Skaha Beach.

*How will I get through this?*

Pond the professional does a quick inventory. Four months sober, no longer craving a drink, yet plagued by persistent and unhealthy levels of anxiety. Mike Pond, the cocky little bastard, has flown the coop, replaced with some pathetic shell of a man wallowing in self-pity.

When it looked like prison was in the cards, Taylor was pitiless.

"This is the result of choices you've made," he said on the phone. "Get some balls."

I'm sober now, but Taylor won't talk to me. I want to make it better between him and me, but I don't even know where to begin. I once asked Dr. Acres why Taylor had cut me out of his life. Dr. Acres didn't say anything, just took a pen, scrawled one word on his notepad and held it up to my face: FEAR. Fear that this period of sobriety will end and the whole crazy cycle will begin again. Fear of answering the phone in case it's the cops telling him I drove drunk again and this time I hit somebody. Or killed somebody. Fear that I'd killed myself. Or worse, that I didn't but I'm thinking about it, again, and he has to talk me out of it, again, but part of him doesn't want to.

Lying here, I have too much time to think. It's so quiet I can't even hear snoring. The bunk below me is empty, a small blessing.

I must find a way to get through this. I need a plan. I repeat the AA slogan: One day at a time; one day at a time. Tim's lady has a place waiting for me when I get out, a tiny attic suite in her old house in White Rock. I am slotted to start work back at Surrey Memorial on January 3, 2010, three days after my release date.

I lie awake that entire first night — nineteen more to go if I get the standard one-third off for good behaviour. And I'm going to be very, very good.

The cell door clicks to signal morning. I slide to the cold floor and peek out into the range. Men exit their cells scratching their heads and crotches. An old inmate pulls the food wagon into the dining area to serve breakfast.

A clean-shaven Lee hands me a plate of fresh toast and peanut butter. The round analogue clock on the far wall reads 8:02 as the thin second hand sweeps across the twelve.

"We're heading for FRCC at nine," says Lee. "We'll go straight to open custody. I'll make sure we get a cell together." Lee always knows what's going on before it happens.

We sit in silence and I force down a piece and a half of Lee's toast, coated with his private stash of peanut butter, a valuable commodity in jail.

A female blue-shirt calls out a string of names. I hear Pond in the mix. Six of us meander to the front desk.

"All of you line up side by side with your noses touching that wall."

We find our spots facing the wall. I smell the old oil-based paint on cinder block and shoot a glance to my left without moving my nose. Three guys down, Lee nods to follow his lead.

"Put your arms straight up over your heads, palms against the wall. Spread your legs shoulder-width apart. Hurry up, let's go! Your right arm behind your back."

While two guards take watch, two others ratchet a set of handcuffs onto our wrists, one click short of too snug. They reach up in unison and pull our other wrists down. Both arms cuffed behind our backs.

"Bend your right leg at the knee," the blue-shirt orders. Shiny shackles ratchet-click around our ankles. "Put it down. Now the other leg."

"Okay, you guys, stand over there by the door and don't move. You other three next." The process repeats. I think back to old prison movies. *Cool Hand Luke. The Longest Yard. The Green Mile.*

We chain-gang single-file out a rear bay door and are greeted by a blast of cold wet delta farmland wind. Even after just one day of institutional air, I gulp its freshness.

"In the vehicle, one at a time, and sit down," says an arm-holstered brown-shirt. The tan paddy wagon interior is pimped out with stainless steel interior wall panels. Heavy-gauge chicken wire reinforces bulletproof glass all around. No blind spots in *this* rig. We perch like wingless redbirds in a cage neatly constructed within an armoured car. The secondary cage door clangs shut. Only Hannibal Lecter could escape this one.

As the armoured van glides off the property, the guards engage in the idle banter that's the talk of free men.

"How 'bout them Canucks, eh?" says the driver.

"Yeah. Luongo couldn't stop a beach ball last night." The brown-shirt sitting shotgun shakes his head in disgust.

"And he's going to be the number one goalie for Team Canada in the Olympics." The driver shoulder-checks onto Highway 1 East. "It should be Marty Brodeur. He's a proven veteran. He's got more experience in Stanley Cup finals."

"And he's consistent. That's what we need — consistency."

The fact that life continues outside prison, that the 2010 Olympics are just a couple of months away, that people are shopping for Christmas presents, that my boys will be planning the holiday with their mother — all these facts flash through my mind.

The paddy wagon cruises down the freeway. The driver exits at 200 Street, Langley. One of my fellow jailbirds observes, "Hey, we're taking the new Golden Ears Bridge to Maple Ridge."

The brand-new bridge spans the mighty Fraser River. I

stare out the window and take it in as we drive over. To the southeast I spot majestic Mount Baker across the border. As my eyes move west toward Vancouver, I recognize Maple Ridge. The small river mill towns of Haney, Maple Ridge and Pitt Meadows now sprawl together into a connecting string of malls, car dealerships and the grand homes of commuters.

I see the Pitt Meadows airport and pinpoint the exact location of my ex-in-laws, the boys' grandparents. They'll all celebrate Christmas there in a couple of weeks. My boys will be there with their cousins and all the rest of the extended family. I always roasted and carved the turkey. I made my special gravy. Many years ago the kids nicknamed me Captain Gravy. Who will be Captain Gravy now?

Within minutes, the van turns left off the mountain road into a large cleared area with manicured, frost-covered lawns. A massive six-storey beige brick structure sits awkwardly in the middle of the clearing. Thirty-foot-high heavy caging encircles the property. Large coils of razor wire crown the cage. Spotlights and all-weather scanning cameras are strategically mounted in every direction.

"Welcome to the joint, boys," says Lee. We pull into Fraser Regional Correctional Centre and the van stops at the bay doors. As the main door unlocks, guards release our shackles, remove our handcuffs and march us into a holding cell. We stand there just a moment while the holding cell door opens and two other young men stumble in.

"Hey, ol' man. How's it goin'?" chirps a handsome grinning dude, about six foot four and twenty-three years old.

"Holy shit! Jarred! How are you, son?" Lee and his son hug and slap each other's backs. Lee's eyes well up and redden. "I can't believe it."

Both of Lee's sons are in prison. Twenty-year-old Lonnie is into his second year of a six-year sentence at Matsqui for aggravated assault — drug deal gone bad.

"This is Mike," says Lee to Jarred. "Fifty-six and he's never done time before. He has three boys about your age, Jarred."

"Nice to meet you, Jarred," I say. "Quite the place for a family reunion, eh?"

"Yeah, crime is a family trait for us Williamses," Jarred nods. "My grandpa started us off, I guess. He did a lot of time in the sixties and seventies, eh, Dad."

Addiction is also a family trait for the Williamses. Clearly, incarcerating three generations did not convince anyone to kick his habit. My clinical brain kicks in once again, and I see these next twenty days in FRCC as a unique opportunity: a living laboratory, if you will. How many of my fellow inmates are here as a result of an addiction?

"Williams, Pond, come with me," orders a blue-shirt as she unlocks the cell door.

"See ya, Jarred. I'll be out December twenty-ninth." Lee waves goodbye.

Once again, we are led down a corridor around a corner to a setup with a large counter facing three open shower stalls. The guard orders us to strip and shower.

Our pants and shirts are bright orange with FRCC stencilled in white on the back. We wear white socks and low-cut, no-name white canvas runners that close with two little Velcro straps. No laces here. Laces make good garrotes — extremely effective at cutting off the airway.

Lee and I step into an elevator. I'm almost getting the routine. Up three floors, the door glides open. Another wide hallway, and an unseen voice directs us via speaker.

The range is big, like in the movies. There are two tiers in the unit, with ten cells per floor — a set of bunks in each, forty men when full. Men sit at square tables playing crib and big two, a long-standing prison card game. There's a TV room. And behind the correctional officers' desk, a large communal shower.

"Hey, man, come over here." An inmate in charge of laundry hands us some folded clothes. "Here's some T-shirts and pants. You get two of each, and keep the ones you're wearing. A couple of long-sleeved thermal undershirts and some work socks. It gets cold in the yard. You'll be working outside in a day or two."

I climb the stairs to the second tier. I've been assigned the first cell, number twelve. An open mezzanine looks out over the range. Several men lean on the railing and look down. I peek into the tiny cell. A young First Nations man with a long braid sits cramped at the desk facing the two-by-three-foot window, bars bolted to the outside. He turns in his chair to face me.

In a low, deep whisper he says, "My name's Nelson. Welcome to my sweat lodge. The guy that left this morning didn't like Indians."

Well, I like Indians, a lot. My work with the Okanagan First Nations makes me Nelson's ideal roommate. Acne scars pockmark his face. He scans me from toe to head. "You're in pretty good shape for an old white man."

"Thanks. My name's Mike." I offer my hand. Nelson's hand has thick, stubby fingers that are slightly webbed. His grip is tight.

"I have a cousin Mike in Kamloops," says Nelson. "He doesn't look anything like you, though. Hahaha!" His too-small eyes are wide set, with no fold in the lid. His forehead is high and broad. He has no indent above his very thin upper lip, all tell tale signs of fetal alcohol spectrum disorder. He's yet another inmate whose life has been defined by alcohol, even before he was born.

A sketchpad sits open on the desk. An orange HB pencil rests ready in his left hand. An exceptional detailed drawing of a naked woman, gagged and tied in bondage, stares up at me.

"Nelson, you've got some talent." I gesture to the sketchpad. "Why are you in here?"

"I beat a guy up on Hastings and Main. I curbed him. He stole my crack."

"I see you got the bottom bunk. I'll put my stuff up here. Talk to you in a bit."

As a therapist in the Okanagan, I've seen first-hand the ravages of alcohol. Fetal alcohol spectrum disorder is rampant on reserves. The physical impairment is mild, the mental impairment devastating: impulsivity, impaired judgment, attention deficits, limited sense of cause and effect. In my two decades of working with the Okanagan bands and my previous experience providing therapy in prisons, I've never known incarceration to act as a deterrent to anyone with a fetal alcohol diagnosis. My empathy for Nelson overrides my self-pity. I am out of here in twenty days. Nelson will likely spend most of his life in places like this. Not because he's an inherently bad man, but because he's been damaged by alcohol.

I leave the cell and walk down the steps to the range. Lee studies a commercial coffee maker that gurgles and spits on a small table, flanked by two four-slice industrial toasters. These and Asian rice makers are highly valued small appliances in the Big House.

"This isn't real coffee," says Lee. "It's chicory or some shit. Jail coffee. We'll have to buy real coffee with our canteen. We put our orders in tonight. You put money in your account, didn't you?"

Some experienced convicts in the recovery house said I would need money to buy necessities. Grant lent me forty bucks yesterday just before we went into court. I had twenty-eight of my own, leftover from my welfare cheque. I put it all in my corrections account when I came in.

"Go over the list," says Lee. "Check off coffee, choneys" — chocolate bars — "chips, soya sauce, curry powder and Asian hot sauce. Buy ten phone calls to start this week. It costs ninety cents for every call, and they add up fast."

I pour a coffee and sit in the TV room with Lee and several other guys. You can tell which guys have been here a while. Their hair is either long or sheared close to the skull. I need a haircut but couldn't afford one before court. I feel old in here. There are a lot of Asians, First Nations and East Indians. White guys are the minority. A guy with snow-white hair down past his shoulder blades, both arms covered with tattoos of pot plants, sits in the corner and watches the Canucks–Kings game. He is the only one close to my age. Early sixties, I estimate.

"How long you get?" he asks.

"Thirty days."

"Sixty. Grow op. I'm Norm," he says.

The dinner wagon rattles onto the range. Convicts line up. Two young Asians serve up the food and fluids. I notice several rice makers on plastic chairs plugged into various outlets in the cinderblock wall. I am second-last in line, with Norm. As each man grabs a tray, select inmates take their baked ham to a couple of other Asians sitting at table nearby. A pile builds, and they proceed to cut the ham into bite-sized pieces with tiny white plastic knives. They deposit the meat into a rice cooker. It sizzles and a head-shaved Vietnamese man dumps a quarter-bottle of sweet hot sauce into the cooker. Close my eyes and I'm in Chinatown, the air redolent with exotic smells.

The men line up at the other rice cookers and another Asian scoops out perfect steamed rice onto each plastic plate.

His cooking partner layers the sweet, spicy, stir-fried processed ham on the bed of rice.

I finally get my tray and look for Lee. There he is, his back against a wall, tray in hand. He scans the dining area. He beckons me over with a jerk of his head. I zero in on a table of several men with two empty seats. Lee follows my line of vision and shakes his head vigorously.

I sit down with three East Indian men who are scooping up hot spicy ham. Two concentrate on their food. The other one peers under heavy black eyebrows in my direction, but somewhere beyond me. He grins without opening his lips. I turn my head and a very large, heavy, muscled Middle Eastern guy sneers down at me. "What the fuck you doing in my seat, old man?" he growls. "Who told you to sit here? You lookin' for fuckin' trouble?"

Somewhere in the deep recesses of my mind I hear, "Ya lookin' fer trouble, lil man? Well ya got 'er right 'ere mister. Come on, git yer dukes up."

In a flash, I'm catapulted back to 1961, Canadian Forces Base Hemer in Germany, where my dad is stationed as a mechanic. Dad loved to play-box with us. I'm glad I paid attention, because I fear those skills are about to come in handy.

Dad's fists came up frequently in a perfect poster-pose, Rocky Marciano–like. "Yer gonna be nuttin' but a greasy spot on da floor when I'm done witch ya," he'd say. "Come on, le's go. Le's go."

Roger and I, six and seven and a half years old, would get our dukes up and dance around shadow-boxing each other, imitating Dad — "Ptew, ptew." Dad would laugh and laugh.

"Come on, Cassius Clay. Let's go, Sonny Liston. Keep those elbows in. Body shots will kill a man. Rupture yer spleen."

I'd be thinking, "What's my spleen? What's a rupture?"

All I knew, it must not be good. So I'd draw my elbows in tight and keep my chin down until it almost cut my airway off. One time Rog accidentally clunked my jaw with a nicely thrown right hook. It stung and shocked me. Then the fight was really on. I nailed him hard with an uppercut and he flew back, landing on the floor sitting up, his arms braced behind his back. His eyes big, he started to cry. Dad stepped in and broke it up.

But Dad is not here today. Real fear grabs me. Two officers watch in silence.

"Sorry, I didn't know," I say.

Lee, with urgency now, says, "Mike. Over here."

I slink over to Lee. We sit together at a table with another new guy.

"You can't sit at a convict's table until you get the nod," says Lee. "Those are Surrey GTs. Mean bitches."

I stay put the rest of the evening, playing crib and looking over my shoulder. At 9:30 it's time to lock down for the day. I dread going to that cell. I walk up the stairs and push open the door.

"Hey!" Nelson yells. "Didn't you see the sign?"

Nelson squats on the steel toilet. The door slams shut and I notice a foot and a half of toilet paper tied to the outside handle. The sign.

I lean on the railing as the men head for their houses. I'm learning fast, the hard way. How did this happen to me? I'm in prison. Prison. Living with murderers and rapists. I'm one of them. My arms tremble as I grip the railing. Two guards check the unit twenty feet below. What will wake me up from this nightmare? A quick vault over the rail and it would be done. Head cracked open like an old egg. One more day is almost done, Mike. Eighteen more to go.

"It's okay, man," says Nelson. "You can come in now. Watch for the sign from now on."

The cell is six by eight feet. A small flat-screen TV hangs from the corner above and to the right of the window. From my top bunk, I can see out the window.

I can't sleep. I can't breathe. I can't think. Big snowflakes float silently down from the black sky. I imagine the stars beyond. Nelson's snores are so loud, they reverberate off the walls of the cell. If I had a knife I'd slit his throat. There's the night-shift guard again. Our eyes connect. The nightlight is too bright. Don't murder a murderer, Mike. Nelson has a mental disorder. He doesn't belong in jail. He belongs, like the majority of the population here, in treatment.

I wait all night for sleep. Nelson's snoring is like the throaty drone of a WWII Spitfire fighter plane climbing into the clouds, up, up, up. Then the silent stall at the peak and the whining whistle of descent. Then up again. Over and over.

Finally, the cell door clicks. I get up and slip out onto the mezzanine, down the staircase to the range, and spot Norman making coffee — real coffee. This smell is not chicory. If I close my eyes, I'm in Starbucks.

"First night in FRCC," says Norm. "How'd you sleep? Without my cannabis, I can't."

"Nelson is a serious snorer. I wanted to murder him in his sleep."

"You fit right in here, then. You going on work detail today?" Norm hands me a mug of coffee.

"Didn't know I was supposed to." I sip my coffee.

"Talk to the guard over there. Tell him you want to start working today. You make $2.75 a day. $13.75 a week. Makes the time go quicker."

The work crew is led down the elevator to the main floor at the back of the institution, where big bay doors accommodate shipping and receiving. One at a time, we strip and get searched and file into a changeroom. The room is stocked with orange overalls, bulky waterproof winter coats and work boots. I'm wearing my thermals. Two corrections officers shepherd us through the secure yard to a large white warehouse. A guy in civvies flies around the yard in a forklift, moving stacks of wooden pallets. There are ten workstations set up throughout the warehouse. Everywhere you look, wooden pallets are piled to the rafters.

A guard says, "Pond, you work with Tremblay. His work partner got released yesterday. He'll show you what to do."

I can see my breath in the fluorescent-lit warehouse air. Tremblay hands me a pair of work gloves. With a thick French Canadian accent he says, "You will need these. In an hour and a half or so, we will take a break and sit under those big heaters and have coffee." He points his gloved finger to the far end of the building. "My name is René."

René demonstrates how to assemble the pallets by arranging the boards in a pattern. We stand facing each other on either side of the pallet form, which sits about waist high. We each hold a pneumatic nail gun. I grab my Makita, one of the best you can buy. René assembles the frame, laying precut two-by-fours into the form. In tandem, we space one-by-fours and fire nails in quick succession. We flip the fledgling pallet over and finish it off with three one-by-fours along the bottom. Because I'm a greener, the job is clumsy at first. But within fifteen minutes, René and I are in sync and assembled pallets fly off the worktable.

An hour and a half in, René says, "We got more than twice as many made than I did with the other guy. He was here three days. Got busted making brew in his cell. Shipped to maximum this morning. Let's go have a coffee."

Despite the fast pace, I'm still chilled. The chicory coffee is hot. With lots of sugar and whitener, it's closer to okay. I don't care. The work has helped me get out of my head, and the time passes more quickly.

Back at the workbench, I pull on my gloves and snug the orange toque over my ears. I reach for my nail gun and bang a three-incher into the wood. The nail head still sticks out of the one-by-four. I slam it down again harder — same results. Three more rapid tries.

"What the hell!"

René keeps his head down, taking over where my nails failed. I notice the nail gun in my hand — it's a yellow Bostitch, a lesser-quality gun.

"Hey! Where's my Makita?"

Without looking up, René's eyeballs roll sideways across the warehouse to land on another workstation. Norm and another guy in a toque, with his back to me, bang away at a pallet.

I pop the Bostitch off the air hose, about-face and march over with it hanging against my thigh. Buddy wearing the toque has my gun. He looks up and stops nailing. It's Raj, the East Indian gangster whose seat I took at dinner. He glances at his gun in my hand, then our eyes lock. His are black and unwavering.

Come on, Cassius Clay. Let's go, Sonny Liston. Keep those elbows in. Body shots will kill a man. My old man's voice fuels my fool's courage. I will not back down.

As Norm cringes and steps back, I step forward. "That's my gun." I feel the pulse pounding in my neck. The fight-or-flight response fully activated, I stand my ground.

"Fuck you, old man! It's mine." Raj is huge, with a blue-black tear tattooed on his left cheekbone. I am told this signifies that he has killed a person. He fires off a few more nails into his pallet.

"I've been using it all day. I'm not leaving till I get it back."

Norm's head swivels back and forth. Raj, then me. Me, then Raj.

On the periphery, several men stop what they're doing.

The bang and buzz of the warehouse slows and dies off. Two guards standing outside the office glance over and stop their conversation.

Expectation hangs in the air. I feel all the blood drain from my head and flood into my arms and legs. My fists clench. All good sense evaporates. I won't throw the first punch — but I'll deliver a powerful second. And then I'll get killed. But what a way to go. There's some dignity in standing up for yourself as opposed to falling down drunk.

A few more seconds of loaded silence pass. Raj's face softens and something resembling respect appears in it. He removes the Makita from the air hose and tosses it on his worktable in front of me. Wordlessly I walk over and hand him the Bostitch.

Walking back to my workstation, I fight the impulse to look back.

"You've got balls, old man," Raj hollers after me.

Maybe, but right now they're up in my throat.

"You're fuckin' crazy," René finally breathes.

That night at dinner, Raj invites me to his table. I smile, thank him and graciously decline.

Work in the pallet plant picks up the pace. Hour after hour, day after day served. Now I'm at thirteen days — only one week to go. I ease my mind by thinking like the professional I once was. Most mental health professionals believe that treating addiction with incarceration is pure idiocy, the worst of public policy and a colossal waste of hundreds of millions of taxpayers' dollars. But rarely is that belief ever reinforced by first-hand experience. If there is to be a gift, a lesson learned from my twenty days at the Fraser Regional Correctional Centre, this is it: incarceration only makes things worse.

The convict addicts obsessively find ways to smoke in a tobacco-free government environment, sneaking behind pallets to puff. Sometimes I join the men in their tobacco rendezvous. I hate smoke, but I crave camaraderie and conversation.

Cut-up fingers from rubber gloves litter the ground. Hooping is happening here. But I shut my mouth.

# 32

# CHRISTMAS

December 24, 2009. Christmas Eve. Five days to go. I have two calls left on my account. I will make one to Rhonda's parents and one to my mother. My mother cries every time I call. How did her son, the little man-child she'd leaned on the most, end up in prison at Christmas? I feel her anguish through the phone. She tries hard to be supportive, but I hear depression and numbness in her voice.

"Just hang in there, Michael," she says. "You'll be out soon. Remember, you have a place and a job to go to when you get out."

I hang on to the knowledge that I have a home when I am released. Tim and his girlfriend will rent me their suite. And, miraculously, I have my job at the hospital waiting for me.

I call Rhonda's parents. They want to come and visit, but I say no. I don't want anyone to see me in this place. I look down at the garb I wear. Normally, red is my favourite colour. Not anymore.

Two of my sons are at their grandparents' for Christmas. Their ladies are with them. I haven't even met Taylor's yet. They have been together for a year. Rhonda is there with her new partner. They are a stone's throw away from FRCC in Pitt Meadows. They might as well be a million miles away.

Christmas day, only four more days to go. Many of the men receive visitors. I don't want any. There are two inmate phones attached to pillars at each end of the open range. I use the one closest to my cell most times. I call my youngest son, Jonny at his grandparents' home. No privacy. Men mill about continually. Swearing. Laughing.

"How's it going, Dad?" Jonny's voice is flat.

"It's going okay, Jon. A few more days and I'll be out. Merry Christmas."

"Merry Christmas, Dad. I'll meet you at the McDonald's in Maple Ridge for a bit when you get out on the twenty-ninth."

"I would really like that, Jon. I haven't seen you since you and Brennan visited in May. How about Taylor?"

"Naw. He's not going to come. I asked him again today. Grandma and Grandpa tried to talk to him, but you know Taylor."

"It's okay, Jon. I know it's hard for him. It's hard for all of you. I'll call you when I get to McDonald's. It'll be mid-morning sometime."

I go back to my cell and lie there, willing the seconds, hours and minutes of an intolerable day away.

Just a few more days to go. I keep my nose clean, do my own time. A group of guys, including me, are being escorted to the gym, when I'm called back to the doctor for a checkup.

I wait at the elevator. The doors open. A guy lies prostrate on the floor, blood gushing from his mouth, as three other men huff and puff and shove past me off the elevator. I rush to tend the collapsed man. "Are you all right?"

"I'm fuckin' all right," he gasps. "Leave me alone." He gets up and hauls himself away.

December 29, 2009, release day. The usual fitful night. I

confirmed on the phone last night that three of my AA friends will pick me up. All I can think about is seeing Jonny.

I take my last elevator ride in Fraser Regional Correctional Centre. I enter the gate admission area, where I arrived nineteen days ago. The white-shirt at the desk hands me all my belongings. I feel stupid as I pull on the old suit. The shoes hurt my feet. I sign my release form and the officer hands me an envelope. I open to find my wallet and $17.75 in cash, a week and a half's wages earned in jail. Thank God for the pallet-plant job.

I scan the parking lot outside. The AA guys have not arrived to pick me up yet.

"Pond, you have fifteen minutes then we release you," an officer says. "Do you want me to phone you a taxi?"

Two other convicts stand dressed and waiting. A taxi arrives.

"Pond, go with these guys," says the officer. "Otherwise you'll be standing out there with no ride into town. Do you need a transit pass?"

I grab the pass and walk out the gate of FRCC for the last time. I am concerned about my ride. Where are they? Maybe Jonny can give me a ride to White Rock.

The two convicts in the taxi chatter about their immediate "discharge plans." Their "corrections aftercare." "I'm goin' straight to my dealer," says one. The other fingers his release cash.

"I'm picking up a forty-pounder of rye — Crown Royal, dude."

Funny. The last thing on my mind is a drink. The taxi pulls up to the bus loop — where the AA guys pull up too. I climb into Grant's van and we head to McDonald's.

As we drive back toward town, I cherry-pick the most entertaining tales from my experience. The guys shake their heads and laugh. Within minutes, we arrive at the

McDonald's. We go in and I sit by the window, looking west. I stare up the street. Tim buys me an Egg McMuffin meal with coffee.

Where is Jonathan? Finally, thirty-two minutes later, at 10:14, Jonny's black Ford F150 pulls into the parking lot.

He gets out and my heart leaps. My throat constricts and I fight back the urge to cry. He hasn't changed a bit since I saw him over seven months ago. Tree Trunk, Big Jon — he's short like his dad, but much thicker. Strong. Sturdy. Solid. And, paradoxically, gentle, kind and compassionate.

He comes in, sees me and smiles cautiously. It's awkward. I don't know what to say.

"Hey, Dad. How are ya?" Jonny stands by our table. "You look pretty good. Kinda thin, though."

I get up and motion Jonny to another table so we can chat alone.

"I'm okay, Jonny." We sit down. "Just happy to be outta there. How was Christmas? How's Grandma and Grandpa?"

"Everybody's good, Dad. Christmas was fine. I'm going back to work New Year's Day."

We chat for half an hour about everything and nothing. His presence is heavy, his sadness a burden almost too much to bear. Who wants to meet their dad coming out of prison at Christmastime?

The AA guys interrupt. "We have to go, Mike," Grant says gently.

But no, I want more, he's just gotten here. But no — I don't think Jonny can hold it together for much longer.

We all walk out to the parking lot together and I give Jonny a hug. I can barely fit my arms around his thick chest and shoulders.

"I love you, son." I squeeze him harder.

"I love you too, Dad." Jonny steps back. "I'll see you later, okay? I'm not sure when." He climbs into his truck and pulls out with a quick glance back and a nod.

I grip the handle on Grant's van to hold myself up. I fight a wave of nausea and the need to collapse. Tears trail down my cheeks. God, what have I done to my boys?

Grant takes the exit and we drive over the Golden Ears Bridge. I gaze west again. I see Pitt Meadows in the near distance. The grey snow-filled sky obscures the view. I imagine my family having lunch at the big kitchen table, chattering and laughing. I'm sure that's Jonny's truck pulling into the driveway now. I can just see it.

# 33

# LIFE GOES ON

January 1, 2010, dawns dark and cold and wet and rainy. I'm back in White Rock, in my new attic apartment. My seventy-seven-year-old mother paid half my rent. She wrote the three-hundred-dollar cheque directly to my landlord, to ensure I had somewhere to go after prison and, of course, to make sure I didn't have the opportunity to drink it.

I paid the other half with the money I'd saved from my last Surrey Memorial paycheque back in August.

I return to work as planned. My new program is work, debt repayment and random urinalysis. Every second Friday, Fraser Health Authority deposits anywhere from $1,400 to $2,000 into my bank account, depending on how much overtime I work. All but the $600 for rent goes to pay down my drunk-incurred debt. One by one, I methodically work through my long list of creditors, paying what I can, negotiating reduced amounts when I can't.

I miss my close-knit group of guys up in Penticton.

I believe I've conquered addiction. It's the loneliness that devours me now.

I miss mountain biking, the grind up Puke Hill with Jim and our wild descent down Campbell Mountain. I miss our pickup hockey games, shooting the perfect tape-to-tape pass right to Alan, who snaps it into the top right corner as Paul the goalie sprawls in defeat, craning to see the puck behind him in the net. I miss going for beers and nachos at the Lakeside. I miss snowboarding down Apex Mountain, carving the champagne powder with Alan and our boys. I ache for my old life. I wonder why they don't call. But I know.

My assignment at work today is to sit and monitor a severely psychotic patient. Wong is just sixteen and borders on brilliance, but he's so mentally ill, there's little chance for it to shine. He has been catatonic for several days — completely unresponsive to any and all stimuli. We query a conversion reaction, which means the patient is in this state but there's no neurological or biological explanation for it. He now requires constant observation.

Here I am desperate for any human interaction, and the one person I'm attending to today can't speak.

"Wong, how are you today?"

"Wong, can you hear me?"

"Wong, would you like a drink of juice?"

Nothing.

I grab his thumb and squeeze hard on the nail bed. I run my pen up the sole of his bare foot. I poke his arm with a sterile needle.

Nothing.

He urinates in the bed again. Mark and I change his wet pyjamas and linens and give him a bed bath. Mark leaves and it's just Wong and me again. He is completely still.

Inexplicably, I'm suddenly gripped by suffocating anxiety. These periods pounce when I least expect them. I try to self-talk my way back to control. I am alone. No one can see or hear me. An involuntary guttural noise escapes from me. This throaty grunt eases the angst. I do a quick scan of the room. No one's coming. No one can hear me. That's good. I allow it to get a little louder. Then a wee bit louder still.

Then, in slow motion, like a corpse coming alive in the

morgue, Wong sits up erect and opens his eyes in an empty stare. He looks directly at me and says, "Would you please stop making that annoying noise." His eyes close and he lies back down.

I snap out of self-absorption. In shock, I pause, then laugh nervously.

An ever-so-slight grin comes over Wong's mouth and disappears just as quickly.

"Mark. Mark." I call out. "Come here. Wong's okay."

Wong's okay, but me — that's a different story.

As the one-year anniversary of my sobriety approaches, August twenty-third, I experience a fresh dread. I've never made it a year. Not even close. I've always screwed up. But something is different this time. I never crave booze. I crave people.

I've been to many one-year cake ceremonies at AA. These are happy affairs, with family and friends and little children running around making a racket. Mine will not be. Outside of a few stalwart AA supporters, it's bound to be a lonely celebration. I text all three of my boys and invite them to the ceremony. Only Brennan, my middle son, drives down from the Okanagan to attend. Surprisingly, or maybe not so surprisingly, my ex-in-laws, Armond and Doreen, deeply religious and compassionate people, smile and take seats.

The usual Fiver meeting has about seventy-five people attend, most of whom I don't know. Some lounge around the long centre row of collapsible tables. Others line around the outside perimeter, their chairs against the wall.

Rotten Randy is here. He walks over, gives me a card and says, "Congratulations. I'd never have dreamed or believed you'd make a year."

Dumbfounded, I mumble my thanks. Throughout my ordeal, especially in the recovery houses, I'd categorized people into good guys or bad guys. But every once in a while someone does something completely out of character. I heard, for example, that Eli from Fresh Start goes to meditation retreats. Who are the villains, who are the heroes? I don't know anymore.

A few of the guys recount Crazy Mike's repeated relapse stories, shaking their heads in wonder that I've finally, finally stayed sober for a year. They are sombre. There is no sense of celebration here, just dogged commitment on their part as AA members to stand by me.

Brennan addresses the group. "I'm glad my dad is sober," he says. He isn't normally at a loss for words, but this simple sentence expresses all that matters.

Then Armond. "Mike has done a lot of bad things," he says to the group. "He's hurt my daughter and grandsons terribly. Sometimes I wanted to hit him. But I still love him and still care about him. Mike is a good man."

Armond's words transport me back to a summer night so long ago when he and I, his wife and my new wife, his daughter Rhonda, went swimming in a small lake in southern BC. A full moon shimmered on the water, activating the phosphorescence. As we glided through the water, our breaststrokes broke the surface and the phosphorescence pushed ahead scattered out of our way like a million fireflies. There was so much magic, so much promise in that night. How could it have all turned out so wrong?

I should feel proud of this accomplishment — sober for one year. Maybe some day I will. But this day is more a crushing reminder of what's lost.

And after the meeting, another loss — young Rob has "gone out." The guys from Mission Possible tell me last they heard he was living under the Granville Street Bridge. Young Rob, who got up at five a.m. to drive me to work, who helped me collect bottles for precious bus fare. Who scrounged the ingredients to make my last birthday cake. Without him, I'd never have made it a year. How will I ever thank him now?

## 34

# THE PRODIGAL
# FATHER

As summer slips into fall, Mark from the Adolescent Psych Unit invites me to join them at the gym. Jim asks me to play tennis. The ordinary invitations stop me in my tracks. I have not done anything like this in years. Nervously, I agree, but wait for them to cancel. I've lived so long with disappointment and rejection, it has become my default setting.

If I'm going to start going the gym or playing tennis, I need runners. I still wear a pair that had been donated to Mission Possible almost a year ago. Having been homeless, penniless and on welfare, I panic when it comes time to parting with money — strange behaviour from a guy who once thought nothing of dropping a hundred thousand on a boat. I can't get my head around indulging myself in a pair of Adidas, half price at sixty-five bucks. A great bargain. I go to the store three times and try them on. I look down at my feet in wonder, because I never thought I'd see the day when I'd be able to purchase my own shoes again. I agonize over the purchase. I finally relent and buy them. Then, wracked with guilt and worry, a week later I return them.

I settle into the idea that I don't have any control over

whether or when my sons will be fully back in my life. Their absence is a chronic dull ache, but I move inexorably toward a new life, where I believe there will some manner of acceptance. I can already feel it.

In just a few days, it will be my fifty-seventh birthday, about a month after my first AA birthday. I am lying on the bed in my attic suite, mentally calculating how much remains on each of my debts, when the phone rings. It's likely a creditor, maybe the hospital asking me to clock an extra shift. I'll call them back.

But that someone just keeps calling and I get irritated. Finally, I crawl off the bed and glance at the number display.

And then I look again. It's a call I've been expecting for two years, and now I'm terrified to answer the phone. Expectation, hope and fear all flood my chest and flush up the side of my face. I pick up the phone.

"Hello, Tay," I say tentatively.

"Dad," he says, his voice heavy with emotion, "I'd like to come and see you."

I hold back the urge to scream out loud, *Yes!* and say, "That would be awesome, Taylor. When do you think you'd come?"

"I'll be in Vancouver this Saturday. I'd like to get you something for your birthday. Take you out for dinner or something."

"You don't need to get me anything. It's enough just to see you, son."

The tears run down my face and I clear my throat to sound unaffected. "See you Saturday."

I count down every hour, minute and almost second until he arrives, on time. That's my Tay, always on time. He pulls up in a brand-new black Dodge Ram 1500 Sport. He's been away working as a lineman apprentice. He climbs down from the truck and just stares. We nervously take each other in.

Taylor is big and burly and handsome, still with that head of curls that makes the girls swoon. I'm thinner, still frail from last year's illness. I fight the tears. My drinking laid waste to his late teenage years. He was his mother's rock and played surrogate father to his younger brothers. What should have been the last carefree years of his youth were spent cleaning up after a drunk, wresting car keys from me or physically kicking me out of our house.

We drive to the pier at White Rock and walk together, our silence interrupted by my rusty, shaky attempts at Dad's humour.

Taylor stops me.

"Dad, I can't do this anymore," he says. "I don't want to be angry anymore. It's not helping me. Or you. Or anyone for that matter. I need to forgive and move on." He smiles. "Happy birthday, Dad."

He wants me back in his life. He wants to forgive me. This nightmare — living a life without what I value most, my sons, has come to an end.

# 35

# SPIRITUAL ENLIGHTENMENT

With Taylor back in my life, I ramp up my recovery. In spite of my ongoing ambivalence about AA, I decide to finish Step 5: admit to God, to ourselves and to another human being the exact nature of our wrongs. Regardless of whether I believe it was the AA program that got me sober, this seems like the right thing to do. But I must find someone who will listen while I confess. Really — who has that kind of time on their hands?

Other men in AA who've done their Step 5 urge me to seek out Sister Monica. They speak of her in hushed tones of awe, respect and gratitude. She and Father Larry run a treatment program just off Vancouver's Downtown Eastside, Bountyfull House.

Sister Monica greets me at the door of Bountyfull House. She's a small woman in her early seventies, with a big, beatific smile. I follow her up the narrow staircase of the rickety old house to one of the small bedrooms, converted to an office.

As I reveal the results of my "searching and fearless moral inventory," Sister Monica listens with absolute compassion and all sense of time and place disappear. She just keeps smiling.

Failures are often judged harshly, especially in recovery houses. Whoever had picked up, gone out or whatever else we chose to call it, was the number one subject of gossip. Some expressed genuine concern and regret for the fellow who relapsed. Others expressed a grim satisfaction, with comments like "I knew that fucker didn't have the balls to see that through." Even our leaders spoke that way.

Five hours after I begin, my Step 5 is complete. I should be exhausted and so should she. But there is a unique energy in the room, born of a sense of fresh possibility.

Sister Monica invites me down to tea with her and Father Larry.

"You've got to take this experience as a gift," Father Larry says to me. To that, Sister Monica adds, "To teach you how to be better at what you do, that is why this happened to you."

I leave the little house on Heatley Avenue light and free.


"Welcome, everyone," says the terminally gorgeous yoga instructor.

What the hell was I thinking? Here I stand, a small, scrawny, past-middle-aged man in spandex shorts, surrounded by real goddess women in my first Bikram Yoga class. After the spiritual cleanse delivered by my Step 5 with Sister Monica, I find myself drawn to the notion of an actual physical cleanse. I've been athletic my whole life and miss the exhilaration of physical exertion. Young colleagues at work rave about hot yoga. So I thought I'd give it a try.

"Do we have any newcomers?" the instructor asks, scanning the room.

The room is so hot, I want to bolt and throw up. But her eyes lock on mine, and I sheepishly raise my hand. No escaping now.

"Hi, my name's Mike and I'm an alcoholic" nearly tumbles out of my mouth. Instead, I say a shy "hi."

"Follow my instructions," says the instructor. "If you feel nauseous or like you may faint, just lie on your back in child's pose or savasana. Please do not leave the room under any circumstances. And try very hard not to drink water until we're through the first series of poses."

Now I really want to bolt.

I fight the nausea and concentrate on following the instructor through a progressively more difficult series of poses. The sweat pours off me. Small puddles form on the hardwood floor and my yoga mat. Rivulets become torrents streaming down my back. I fight for oxygen. A blinding headache forces me to the floor.

As I lie there and collect myself, I imagine running outside to gasp mouthfuls of fresh ocean air. I think back to the sweat lodges I attended with the Okanagan First Nations on the banks of the Similkameen River. I fought similar urges there, too. I remember how transformative the heat could be, how the simple act of just being with the difficulty was in itself a path to spiritual enlightenment.

I stay put. The nausea subsides and so, finally, does the headache. I get up and finish the class. Walking home, the world has an enhanced quality. There is more sparkle to the twinkling lights of the city. With each inhalation, the ocean air crackles. Blood pumps furiously throughout my body. Whatever this drug is, I want more of it.

I walk to the White Rock Bikram Yoga studio every day, sometimes twice a day, and on my days off, three times a day. Typical Mike, who can do nothing in moderation.

A few months into my three-times-a-day hot yoga addiction, my young colleagues at work eye me appreciatively, exchange glances among themselves. And then Jim, obviously designated pitchman, speaks.

"Mike, it's time we put you on Plenty of Fish."

"What's plenty of fish?" I blink at them.

About half a dozen staffers collapse in giggles. Tracey rolls her eyes.

"Internet dating, Mike. Once we take your picture and post your profile, you'll feel like captain of the football team all over again."

After being married for twenty-five years and lost in an alcoholic fog for the last three, I'd missed the Internet dating phenomenon completely. The only email I receive is from Groupon.

Soon, the distinctive ping of email notification punctuates each workday. Dozens and dozens of women appear interested in me. During breaks, my colleagues read each prospective new partner's profile online, pass judgment on the picture and suitability of each respondent, and pick the lucky women with whom I should correspond. And so begins a blissful, giddy period in my life. During each lunch break, I engage in several satisfying email flirtations. Every evening after work, I meet a different woman for coffee.

And the inevitable questions begin. "So why don't you drink? And why aren't you driving?"

"I'm an alcoholic," I explain. "I lost my driver's licence for drunk driving."

I hope that rigorous honesty will impress.

"Thank you. I don't feel the connection."

"Sorry. I don't date men shorter than five foot ten. It's just my thing."

"I love my wine. I don't think it's right to drink in front of you. Good luck. I'm sure there's a wonderful woman out there just waiting for a nice guy like you."

And so it goes. Plenty of Fish serves up an endless conveyor belt of attractive women who clearly do not listen to their mother's admonitions about meeting men on the

Internet. If they only knew half the truth about me, they'd run screaming from the room.

November 21, 2010 — I'm tired from a wicked shift, but I have another Plenty of Fish encounter planned. I almost cancel. The SkyTrain rattles through the city. I'm en route to meet, at rough estimate, my fifteenth first date since I started online dating over a month ago. Maureen and I have talked on the phone a few times.

"I'm a therapist," I said. "I work at Surrey Memorial in psychiatry. My plan is to open a private practice in Vancouver." I don't tell her I have an apartment with absolutely nothing in it but a bed. Buying furniture is not on my debt repayment plan.

She's a former journalist, now a filmmaker. A journalist. Great. She'll take probing to a whole new level. I approach Steamworks Brew Pub. As I approach, I spot an attractive, well-dressed, diminutive middle-aged woman, reaching into her seriously overstuffed purse. She looks up and we immediately recognize each other from our profile pictures. I'm surprised she actually looks like her picture. Now a veteran of Plenty of Fish, I've seen more than a few women seriously underestimate their age and weight.

She's fumbling for change to give to a street fellow with a three-toothed grin. As her big purse slides around on her thigh, a pink curler plops onto the pavement. I will come to understand that neither of these two things — the giving, or the random appearance of pink rollers—are uncommon events.

I also hand the guy a few bucks. "Here you go, buddy."

"Thank you, sir. You're both angels."

There but for the grace of God, go I.

"That was very nice," Maureen smiles. "I have a soft spot for those guys."

Hmmmm. This may go better than I thought. We walk into the bar together and take a table close to the window, overlooking the water and boats. When the waiter arrives, she orders a glass of Chardonnay.

"And for you?"

"Cranberry juice and soda," I say with faux confidence.

"You're not ordering a drink?" Maureen's eyebrows lift. Shit, here we go again.

"I don't drink," I say. Here it comes.

"Why don't you drink?"

When I tell her, she doesn't dash for the door. She seems intrigued, even. We plan another date. And another. Slowly, I unpeel the layers of the onion that is my story. I censor myself. Yes, I was in recovery homes last year, I admit. I'm sober a little over a year.

The night before our second get-together, she says on the phone, "I know my friends would be nervous if they knew about your alcoholism, but I want to tell you Mike, the fact that you're an alcoholic ... it's not a deal breaker. You've been sober more than a year, and I think if you have the courage and discipline to stop drinking, then the least I can do is keep an open mind."

We spend Christmas Eve together in her beautiful condo backed up against Grouse Mountain in North Vancouver. As we sit and cuddle on the couch admiring the twinkly Christmas tree, she absently asks, "Where did you spend last Christmas, Mike, with some of the AA guys?"

"Yes, something like that." I nod. I was in prison, but she can't know that. Not yet. Then of course, she asks the most difficult question of all. "Why did you drive drunk?"

Aside from the turmoil I wrought on my boys' lives, the decision — or rather non-decision — to drive drunk is the aspect of my story for which I feel the most shame. I consider my answer a long time before I respond.

"I drove drunk," I say, "because I was a drunk. As my alcoholism progressed, judgment disappeared. I went through a stage of giving people my keys, to prevent me from driving. Then that got to be too big a burden on people I loved. They stopped taking them. Then, as my condition worsened, my ability to make a reasoned choice disappeared. Nothing can make it right."

That's all I can say. I sense she's disappointed, like she expected something more insightful, something that would allow both of us to let me off the hook a bit.

Over the next few months, I unfold my complete story before Maureen. As I peel back each consecutive layer, her eyes pop even wider. Her body coils as if to pounce. Is this where she says, no more, she's had enough? No — recognizing a good story when she sees one, she bristles with excitement. One night she says, "You have to write a book, Mike."

I write, delete, rewrite and delete. After two weeks, I proudly present Maureen with my twenty-page masterpiece. After a couple of pages, she scrunches her nose, tilts her head sideways and looks at me with a protruding upper lip. "Not bad for a first go round."

I exclaim, "Not bad! I do know how to write, you know."

She tilts her head a little farther, looks me straight in the eye and says firmly, "Listen. Do you want to write a book people will read, or do you want me to blow smoke up your ass?" I think it was that moment I finally fell completely and irrevocably in love with Lil Mo.

I fell in love with her grit and her wit. And more than that, I fell in love with her generosity of spirit. Not just with me, but with everyone. It takes a special person to take the heavy odds against building a relationship with a freshly recovered alcoholic. Maureen is that special person: a risk taker, an adventurous soul. She came into my life at a time when I was just beginning to believe in myself again, and having her believe in me too has enabled me to solidify my recovery, to have the courage to tell my story in this book.

# 36

# I KNOW THAT WALK

Sometimes, much as I hate to admit it, I act like an alcoholic even if I don't crave a drink. On occasion I find myself mired in classic alcoholic behaviour, the behaviour Sigmund Freud characterized as "King Baby." It's an obsessive, intensely self-focused kind of thinking that doesn't leave much room for anyone else. It's my place of resentment, where I coldly calculate my spreadsheet of losses. It doesn't happen often, but the more I engage in it, the more Maureen points out all the amazing accomplishments of my new life. The more she suggests I concentrate on being grateful, the more cranky and pissed off I get.

One spring night, after a few days of dealing with King Baby, Maureen has had quite enough. She suggests we attend the closest AA meeting. Right now. So off we go, in cold silence, to a meeting in North Vancouver, just a few minutes from home.

I walk in ahead of her and she follows, fighting tears of frustration. She won't talk as she struggles to regain her composure. We find two wooden chairs next to the wall and stare ahead as the room fills to capacity. Everywhere around us, members greet each other with warmth and encouragement.

The chair is just about to call the meeting to order. Maureen turns to me, eyes wide.

"That's Dana," she says with certainty. She looks back at a tall woman with striking red hair who is walking into the room, her back to us.

My heart jumps into my throat. I know that walk. I know that hair, pinned up exactly as I remember it. Maureen knows it intuitively now too, because we've been writing this story together. The woman takes her seat immediately across the room from me. Our eyes lock. Dana. Of all the AA meetings in all the towns in the world, she had to walk into mine.

It's been a few years since we've seen each other. She'd call me on occasion, but I rarely picked up, because I know how dangerous Dana and I can be together.

My hands tremble as I remember the wild ride over Naramata Road that landed us in jail. The two of us staggering to the liquor store the next morning. Dana buying me winter clothes so I could survive on the street. Breaking into her friend's house and drinking every drop in sight. Springing me from Fresh Start. The many times her convertible Miata sped off into the night, her long red mane flowing behind her in the wind. Dana, sitting at the end of my hospital bed, slurping Red Bull and vodka as I hovered near death. Betraying me with Big Stu. Dana, Dana, Dana. The damage we did to each other, and to everyone else who cared about us. I'm mad at her, mad at myself. Relieved she's here because maybe she's finally sober now, too, but unnerved as hell because just when I finally get my act together, here she is again. I wish her well, but I worry what any contact with her will do to me. Will I want her sober? Will she still want *me* sober? What's Maureen thinking now?

The chair begins. "This is an AA open meeting. Could we have a couple of topics please?"

A middle-aged woman calls out, "Humility."

An older gentleman says, "Step 3."

Another man in the back yells, "Gratitude."

"Thank you," the chair says. "That should be enough." His eyes sweep the room fix and fix on mine. I hold his gaze. The non-verbal interaction confirms the invite and consent to speak. He smiles.

"Would you like to share?"

First to share. I get the opportunity to set the tone of this meeting. My head tips left, and I unconsciously scratch that one spot on the crown of my head and my face flushes self-consciously.

"Sure," I pull in a deep breath. "My name's Mike and I'm an alcoholic."

A chorus of "Hi Mike's."

I look directly across from me to see Dana's lips pout and those big blue eyes widen. She shifts in her chair and stretches the fingers of her hand on her knee to inspect her nails. Perfect as always.

I clear my throat.

"This is my first time at *this* meeting and it's good to be here. I've been sober two and a half years and I think my brain is just now starting to function somewhat okay. I lost everything due to my drinking. And now it's all starting to come back. My sons are talking to me again. I am practising my profession again. I'm in an amazing relationship. And I'm very, very grateful tonight."

I gaze sideways at Maureen. Her eyes brim. She's angry now, because all day I refused to be grateful about anything. Now the group nods appreciatively and I bask in their approval and she still thinks I'm a dink.

Dana watches us and crosses her legs. I can't gauge her reaction.

Several more people share. A young man offers, "I ended up almost dead on the Downtown Eastside. I had to surrender my will and get humble. I thank this program for saving my life."

A shudder crawls up the back of my neck as I remember, not so long ago, wandering those same streets, lost and lonely in the black cold rain, panhandling for beer money.

"Thank you." The chair nods. "I think we have time for one more." Once more he scans the room. He stops at Dana.

"Would you like to share, ma'am?"

"Yes, I would. My name's Dana and I'm an alcoholic. I'm three months sober. The whole thing has been very humbling." Dana recounts her humiliations and her triumphs. So, in front of a hundred unaware strangers, we catch up on each other's lives.

After the meeting, Maureen and I stand looking at each other, the question unspoken.

"Go over and talk to her, Mike," Maureen says, and slips out into the hall.

I weave my way over to Dana, neither of us quite able to take in what just happened. How we're actually together after all this space and time, in the same room.

The crowd falls away. I search my heart and the truth pops out of my mouth. "I'm glad you're getting on track, Dana."

Her eyes spark with that familiar fire and I feel myself drawn to her. Oh God, not now, just when I've really got my shit together. She gazes up at me with a look that's part come-hither but more "holy shit, I can't believe we're both standing here sober and alive."

We stand and stare and process. And then I surrender. It's over and we both know it. Romance has taken a back seat to regret. We both have done each other too much harm.

We are at a loss for words. Which is a first for us.

"Take care, Dana."

"Be well, Mr. Pond."

I am.

# THE SEVEN
# QUESTIONS I GET
# ASKED THE MOST

I remember when Dr. Acres said, "It can all come back, Mike. Maybe not the way it was, or how you want it, but it can all come back."

It has all come back. And more. My life revolves around my sons, my relationships and my work. The woman who asked the relentless probing questions was undeterred — we're still together. As of this moment, I am coming up on five years sober and have a thriving new practice in Vancouver. Not surprisingly, many of my clients battle addiction, and they pepper me with questions. These are the most frequent ones.

## 1. "MIKE, WHAT FINALLY GOT YOU SOBER?"

I continue to struggle with a definitive answer to that question. Maybe I just didn't want to die a drunk. I didn't want to leave that legacy for my sons. *But more importantly, I finally wanted to be sober. I wanted to be sober more than I wanted anything else.* More than having my boys back in my life, more than Dana, more than having my job back. And as I lay in that hospital bed in Surrey Memorial, seriously ill with pneumonia, I was forced to confront the very real possibility that

I would die. There's a possibility that twenty-eight days of intensive rest and care reset my altered brain. All I know is the longer I lay in that hospital bed, the more motivated I became to not drink again.

## 2. "BUT YOU MUST HAVE DECIDED TO QUIT DRINKING. SURELY THERE IS AN ELEMENT OF CHOICE HERE?"

I'm not sure about that one. Approximately 80 per cent of people who begin drinking do just fine. But in a sizable minority of us, alcohol flicks some kind of switch that causes an array of neurotransmitters in our brain to run amok.

Marc Lewis, author of *Memoirs of an Addicted Brain*, says, "I *don't* see addiction as a disease. I do see it as changing the brain, as do other developmental phenomena, like learning to talk or falling in love." Lewis doesn't think *disease* is the term to describe addiction. Nor is it a character flaw. Nor is it choice. What it is ... is complicated. And we are just beginning to understand it from a neurobiological point of view. To quote Lewis, "Addicts lose the mental muscle tone for self-direction, for resolve, for strength of character, and for decency itself." Lewis believes addiction is an altering of the brain: one that can be repaired. There's also growing proof that faulty genetics plays a big role in this.

I think addiction is an amalgam of all this – part brain disorder, part genetics, part learned behaviour, part self-medicating and in some individuals, part choice.

I think addiction, or whatever you choose to call it, actually robs some of us of our capacity to make sound choices. Lewis theorizes that the part of the brain that's critical to decision making, judgment, choice and self-monitoring gets tired. It "gets exhausted by the simple act of saying 'no' to temptation." As addicts we're faced with saying "no" every second, every minute, every hour of every day. Then, "there's a loss of flexibility as synapses and habits rigidify. The physical limitations of brain matter itself provide the cause. The breakdown of human functioning is the consequence." This rings truest to me.

## 3. "WHAT KEEPS YOU SOBER?"

At the beginning of my recovery: AA. There's nothing like being with people who get it. I needed to be around people who understood me. In AA, I got the most acceptance, and ironically, the most judgment. The AA model in the Fresh Start Recovery Home and Mission Possible was so shame-based, it made my condition worse. I believe my wanting to get out of those places was my strongest motivation. It shoved me out of a state of ambivalence and fear to a state of self-determination. I became motivated from within. *This is the critical piece.* While addicted, I made all manner of bad choices. As time progresses, addicts grow not to trust our decision-making capacity, for good reason. We then exist in a prolonged state of inertia and ambivalence. To experience motivation after not having it for years is a powerful thing. Looking back, I believe I applied some Motivational Enhancement Therapy on myself.

I now believe the foundation of any treatment program must be evidence-based and from a place of non-judgment and compassion and acceptance.

Back then, the biggest break I got, and kept getting, was from the union representing psychiatric nurses and from the Fraser Health Authority. Both treated my addiction like the disorder it is — and stuck by me when I relapsed not once but twice. Very few people battling addictions get that kind of support. I'm humbled by it to this day.

By year two of recovery, writing this book kept me sober.

It was a form of therapy, writing the narrative, rewriting it over and over, making sense of it. I was essentially using every strategy in my psychotherapy toolkit on myself. Perhaps the intensity of writing built new habits, new neural pathways in my brain, such that I don't crave a drink. Ever.

My relationships keep me healthy now. It's indescribable loneliness that drives many back to the bottle, or worse — to suicide. If it hadn't been for Maureen coming along when she did, if it hadn't been for Taylor's forgiveness, if it hadn't been for Brennan and Jonny being willing to stick with our faltering relationship, I honestly don't know if I'd be here. I also credit Rhonda, my ex, with urging the boys to keep the door open to a relationship with their father. I put her through hell. She has approached my recovery with a generosity of spirit.

## 4. "WHY DID YOU HAVE TO HIT ROCK BOTTOM BEFORE YOU QUIT?"

A lot of people in my life said to my face that I had to bottom out. We've all said it in conversation: "He's one of those guys who has to hit rock bottom." *No one has to hit rock bottom.* That's where I've had one of the biggest paradigm shifts. Think in terms of other illnesses or disorders. The earlier the diagnosis is made, especially in life-threatening conditions like cancer, the better the outcome. With a cancer diagnosis we throw the best, most aggressive treatment at the illness. Addiction kills too, yet we hold on to the anti-quated notion that bottoming out is what the worst of us must do. Bottoming out costs us all too much. I think of what I cost the system — in health care, incarceration, social assistance — and I shudder. And that's not factoring in the greater losses: my relationships, my practice and the personal degradation. I think of all the others like me who never get to realize their potential. Studies now show, as with most mental disorders, the earlier you receive credible treatment for substance use problems, the higher the probability of successful outcome.

## 5. "SO WHAT'S THE ANSWER?"

We need to approach addiction as the life-threatening condition it is. We need to have swift and universal access to mental health and addiction services. The more deplorable recovery homes need to be shut down and all of them must be investigated, licensed and regulated. We need family and friends to get actively involved, and early, from a position not of judgment, but of kindness. And we need the system to support *them*, too. This is not a quick fix. The freshest research on addiction suggests that a long period of positive interactions while gradually weaning the addict from his substance abuse may result in the most long-term success. Yes, this costs money, but untreated addiction costs so much more.

And it will continue to cost us billions, as long as we hold on to attitudes that blame the individual for his addiction. The widely held societal belief that addicts are flawed, "less than," and should be judged harshly, allows the punishment model to flourish. No one would dream of putting a cancer patient in a care centre where rats drop out of the ceiling, where administrators run off and sell the patients' meds on the street, where patients are assaulted at knifepoint, where group leaders and counsellors ridicule and humiliate those who don't get better, where photos of those who succumb to their illness are circled in black. Why do we allow such places to exist by the hundreds in the Vancouver area alone and use the word *recovery* in their names? They are unlicensed, unregulated and mostly unfit for human habitation. We allow it because many of us believe that's what addicts deserve.

## 6. "ALL WELL AND GOOD IN SOME IDEALISTIC FUTURE, BUT WHAT DO I DO WITH MY ADDICTED LOVED ONE NOW?"

First, educate yourself. Blogs like Marc Lewis' and Dr. Gabor Maté's provide fresh and thought-provoking information about the nature of addiction. It's really important to know what the brain research tells us, because it has an impact on how to treat it. We now know for certain that shaming an addict will not help the problem, so any program that involves shaming is not useful. Now, go in search of a therapist who is also up-to-date on addiction theory and practice. Ask pointed questions of the clinician. Make sure you are satisfied with her or his approach before you entrust a loved one to their care.

Second: I understand your frustration and pain, from both sides. From my own experience recovering, I've come to realize addiction is a systemic problem perpetuated by family, community and the world at large. The solution is systemic too. A new guide for families called *Beyond Addiction: How Science and Kindness Help People Change* offers an evidence-based proven alternative to the shame-and-blame model. This book is from the Center for Motivation and Change, which does workshops and trainings in CRAFT — Community Reinforcement and Family Training. More addicts get sober and stay sober when their families support their recovery. This is not just about showing up on family day at the treatment centre. In the CRAFT model, family members are trained to use "positive, supportive, non-confrontational techniques," which help not only the addict, but family members too. Clinical trials have shown that family members benefit emotionally, *even if their loved ones don't go into treatment.*

Finally, we need to force the government to confront one of the greatest public health problems in our country, with compassion — and not by criminalizing us. In my twenty-one days in prison, I did a rough calculation of how many of my fellow inmates were there because of an addiction-related offence: three-quarters. What a waste of resources and lives. Activism has transformed the stigma around AIDS and breast cancer and prostate cancer treatment. Families and friends of addicts and reformed addicts like me need to step up.

## 7. "HOW HAS THIS EXPERIENCE CHANGED YOU?"

As a clinician, I've been humbled. Before my downfall, I thought I did a pretty good job empathizing with my addict clients. But to have personally experienced such profound loss, humiliation and anxiety, and depression so entrenched that suicide seemed a relief, has taught me much more than any graduate degree could. I understand what it feels like to be ridiculed, judged and shamed. Today I truly understand my clients' despair, because I have lived it. I like to say, "Now I *really* know what I'm talking about!"

I've changed too, in some ways I'm not proud of, ways in which I continue to struggle. Having lost everything and experienced rejection on such a grand scale, I went through a period of hypersensitivity to it, especially in areas of my life where I feel vulnerable, like with my boys. On days when I'm stressed, if one of my boys cancels a dinner or a hockey game, I can plummet to the depths of despair, convinced they once again don't want anything to do with me. Such hyper-vigilance to threat kept me alive in prison, in downtown back alleys and in down-and-out recovery homes. As a clinician, I know it evolved for good reason. If a patient came to me with the same problem, I'd help them reframe it positively by saying things like "Quite often, twenty-two-year-olds cancel plans with their parents. How many twenty-two-year-olds do you know who like to hang with their folks?" Because I experienced such hyper-vigilance and fear of rejection, I can address those feelings in my clients much better now.

My colleague at St. Paul's Hospital in Vancouver, Dr. Chris Gorman, puts it another way. He suggests that those who have suffered from mental illness and the addiction often entwined with it are not less than, but *more* than. More than means that they have experienced a breadth and depth of human experience that eludes most. They have been tempered by fire, made stronger, more resilient. This is how I suggest that my clients who battle addiction think of themselves.

These are exciting times in addiction treatment. We've finally tipped over from the "one way fits all" approach to recognizing that science now offers evidence-based research and treatment that have more successful outcomes. But we have a long way to go before this idea has widespread public acceptance. This book is part of my fight to make that happen.

As for myself ... I continue to be a work-in-progress.

# ACKNOWLEDGMENTS

## To my family:

I am grateful to all those who stayed with me through the insanity and loved me when I wasn't very lovable. I am also grateful to those who couldn't stay, especially my son Taylor. The hope of rebuilding my relationship with him one day helped keep me sober. Thank you, Brennan, for always taking my calls and for coming to my one-year anniversary sobriety cake ceremony. Jonathan: for being there the day I was released from prison, thank you.

To my mother and her husband, Paul, there are no words to describe the depth of gratitude I feel toward you. I'm blessed that you are still in my life and I am sober. I love you, mum. I also wish to thank my dad and step-mum Christel, for coming through with cash at the critical moment. To my ex-in-laws, Armond and Doreen, who came to see me in the hospital and in the recovery house: your acceptance was a soothing constant in my life.

To my siblings: Danette, Loretta and Roger, thank you for allowing me to share painful parts of your private lives too.

And finally: Rhonda. Thank you for all the great years and happy times. I am sorry for all the heartache and stress I put you through. As an ex-wife and mother they don't come much better.

# TO THOSE WHO HELPED CREATE *THE COUCH OF WILLINGNESS*:

Trena White and Jesse Finkelstein, who created Page Two Strategies, a new model for ensuring high-quality self-publication in the digital age. Trena is the former publisher of Douglas & McIntyre and Jesse is the former chief operating officer. Their vision, warmth, belief in the story and dedication to detail made publishing this book a gratifying experience.

A huge thank you to Tamara Chandon, of UBC's Booming Ground non-credit creative writing program, who edited our first draft and provided vital feedback and coaching throughout. Tamara, thanks for seeing the potential and believing in it.

To our friends, author Claudia Casper and her husband, James Griffin, and filmmaker Helen Slinger, who read the first draft and told us we'd crafted a page-turner. Your support and deep friendship mean the world to us.

# TO THOSE WHO HELPED ON THE PATH TO SOBRIETY:

I'd love to use your real names: members of Alcoholics Anonymous, doctors, nurses and social workers who never gave up on a drunk, but you know who you are. Thank you.

I can't forget the other drunks, addicts and homeless guys who quite literally gave me the shirts off their backs so that I could get back to work. Rob, who made my birthday cake, who scrounged in ditches for empties so I could raise a week's bus fare, who performed so many selfless gestures ... thank you. Wherever you are, buddy, I wish you peace and sobriety.

To my old friends: Dale Wallace and his wife, Deb, who stuck by me for thirty-eight years. I can never repay your kindness and loyalty. To Brian and Irene and Ralph and Jan and Troy, Derek and Mary, thank you for not turning your backs on me in Penticton. Deb, your deer roasts, and Doug, your sweat lodge on the banks of the beautiful Similkameen River, helped me heal.

I'm very indebted to my clients, past and present, who find solace and inspiration in my story, especially First Nations clients such as Rhonda Terbasket, who stuck by me even when they deserved much better. I'm sorry I couldn't get sober sooner.

To the staff at APU at Surrey Memorial Hospital: you probably had some idea just how fragile I was when I returned to work. Your support ensured I kept my job, which ensured I stayed sober. And then you wrote my profile, took my picture and uploaded it all to Plenty of Fish. You saw my loneliness and took action. You transformed my life.

## To the people in my new life:

New friends: Anne and Tony Giardini, Tony Harrison, Adrienne Tanner and Mike Walker, Sue Ridout and Bruce Mohun. You helped me believe life can be good again.

To Maureen's warm and often wacky family: I so needed to laugh again and you taught me how.

To Maureen, who took quite a chance on a newly recovered alcoholic, I love you.